Keyworking

An examination of a method of individualising care for older people in residential establishments

IAN MALLINSON

Avebury
Aldershot • Brookfield USA • Hong Kong • Singapore • Sydney

Published by
Avebury
Ashgate Publishing Limited
Gower House
Croft Road
Aldershot
Hants GU11 3HR
England

Ashgate Publishing Company
Old Post Road
Brookfield
Vermont 05036
USA

British Library Cataloguing in Publication Data

Mallinson, Ian
Keyworking: Examination of a Method of
Individualizing Care for Older People in
Residential Establishments
I. Title
362.61

ISBN 1 85972 179 6

Library of Congress Catalog Card Number: 95-80346

Typeset by the Central Text Production Unit, Moray House
Moray House Institute
Holyrood Road
Edinburgh

Printed and bound by Athenaeum Press, Ltd.,
Gateshead, Tyne & Wear.

Contents

Figures and tables

Summary

This book explores the question: Does keyworking in residential care for older people contributes towards improved individualised care?

A research agenda was constructed through a review of the themes contained in the literature on keyworking. These themes may be grouped into two areas: relationships and decision making/meeting needs. Following SCA (1991) keyworking is generally seen as 'a system for providing individualised social care through named persons. A keyworker is the person who has responsibility and accountability for the care of the service user and for decisions relating to their situation.' Considerable variations were however found in the way keyworking is defined, and in the ways that practice is interpreted.

A small scale research exploration, was formulated. This established first the context and effect of keyworking through a survey questionnaire administered (as part of a wider census of care practices) to a number of establishments. The research thereafter explored the nature of the practice of keyworkers in individualising care through case study interviews conducted in two individual establishments. Comparisons were made, recommendations and principles for practice developed.

It was found that keyworking in residential care for older people does contribute towards improved individualised care. Keyworking practice was particularly effective when considered within the broader context of group living and the overall work of the staff team. Its effectiveness is, however, dependent upon the calibre of a broad tapestry of systems and structures (in particular those concerning supervision, evaluation and care planning), how these are utilised within keyworker systems and upon the nature of the individual keyworker/ service user relationship. The weakness of the concept lies in the variability of practice and relationships within establishments when minimum standards and requirements are not defined and/or not applied.

1 Introduction

1. The purpose of this book

The concept of keyworking in residential care has not hitherto been subject to academic analysis. Any research has been secondary, exploring keyworking not as an entity but taking it as incidental to and on the margins of other areas of exploration. It is the author's personal experience that keyworking practice is fragmented, there being many different definitions and versions of keyworker systems (often within the same establishment). It could be argued that these variations in practice reflect a notion that keyworking is an idea, not a concept, despite being referred to as the 'keyworker concept' in most of the literature. Keyworking as an idea is a simple formulation ie. that individualised care may be best provided through a named individual. A concept may be seen as a broader complex of objects all of which share the same attributes. There appears to be however a large number of different interpretations and definitions of keyworking practice in existence. The variety of practice that materialises as a result illustrates weaknesses in the formulation, or the possibility that a single formulation does not exist. It can be suggested, that keyworking may mean (to those involved in providing individualised care) all and everything, or may mean little and nothing.

This book is the first time that the nature of keyworker practice in residential care has been researched. Keyworking practice in residential care for older people is a neglected area in academic analysis. Apart from works on other areas of practice (that treat keyworking incidentally to their main subject) accounts of practice are anecdotal and largely descriptive. There are some accounts of theoretical principles but these have not been tested in research or in reports of actual practice.

The central question to be explored in this book is: Does keyworking in residential care for older people contribute towards improved individualised care? For the first time in reported research the context and the nature of keyworker practice in such settings is considered.

The wide variations in practice referred to would appear in the author's experience to be reflected throughout the care sector. In exploring the question whether keyworking contributes towards improved individualised care in residential settings, cognizance needs to be taken of such variations. These variations appear to partially derive from various developments in keyworking during and since the mid/late 1970s.

2. A spectrum of practice types

The first formulation of 'keyworking' was an attempt in 1976 to define roles spanning boundaries between fieldwork and residential care (RCA/BASW 1976). The 'concept' of keyworking/ keyworker systems was based upon consolidation and extension of link roles previously devised between settings in the 1960s. RCA/BASW (1976, 347) thus defined a keyworker as 'the person having full responsibility for the service user received into residential care and for decisions relating to the case.' They elaborated this as covering all stages (pre-admission, admission and rehabilitation) and spanning all the settings then involved (eg. fieldwork and residential care). The keyworker's primary focus here was said to be decision making and co-ordination.

This may now be compared with a contemporary definition for keyworking in social care by SCA (1991). This definition is one which is often used in the social care sector. A keyworker is part of 'a system for providing individualised social care through named persons. A keyworker is the person who has responsibility and accountability for the care of the service user and for decisions relating to their situation.' This version of keyworking links direct, hands on care, with internal decision making in social care and no longer primarily concerns spanning boundaries between settings. This definition, it may be suggested, reflects a large amount of current practice in residential care, and is the definition used in this book.

In residential work keyworking now focuses upon arrangements for individualised care through a named person who is said to be responsible and accountable for the nature of the individual experience. In analysing the nature and effect of this (particularly in relation to evolving systems under the 1990 NHS and Community Care Act) Cambridge (1992) states that keyworking focuses primarily upon day to day relationships. This may be contrasted with keyworking based primarily upon co-ordination in planning (based within settings involving purchasing roles eg. those in care management). Whilst a purchaser/ provider split implies a polarisation of these into two ideal types, in practice it may be that a spectrum of different types exists. Thus keyworking in residential care may be located at the 'relationship' end of the spectrum but may also involve elements of co-ordination.

This book explores individualised care in residential establishments for older people. Keyworking appears to have become a particularly meaningful method of practice as a specialising role (see eg. DHSS, 1979). The bulk of the literature on relationships and individualisation within residential care has, however, been based upon 'armchair theory' rather than upon research. Any exploration of keyworking practice should consider the nature of those formulations and the issues they present for practice.

3. Issues in practice: the rationale for the book

It was SCA/BASW, in an influential but unpublished report of a working group reviewing the nature of keyworking in social care, (1987) who suggested that the keyworker is usually seen as the person who is responsible for the individual care of service users based upon personalised relationships within the context of the group setting. It was from this report that the widely used definition previously referred to (SCA 1991) was later formulated. Here, the internal planning necessary to meet the needs of individuals and groups of service users is often carried out jointly between keyworkers and supervisors.

A large number of writers highlight inflexibility and confusion resulting from a lack of clarity in keyworker systems in residential care (eg. Davis, 1978; and Douglas and Payne, 1980) and the unrealised potential of keyworker systems (eg. Elliott, 1978). The suggestion is made in these works that the role of a keyworker is highly skilled, but often becomes an empty title (eg. Hogan, 1988) and that keyworker systems generally enable greater client choice (but in some circumstances may present many other problems and practice dilemmas, eg. those concerning conflicting values and power; see for example, Davis, 1978; and Mallinson and Best, 1987).

Despite these issues, the influential Barclay report firmly recommended that keyworkers be appointed for every person in day or residential care (NISW, 1982). The evidence in the Wagner report, as a major review of practice, (NISW, 1988) points to extensive implementation, stating that it was seen by some as '... the most significant development in residential care for all client groups' (p 197).

Elkan and Kelly (1991) however, in their important literature analysis of aspects of residential care, summarise the approaches to keyworking in relation to group care as 'essentially individualised responses to the provision of care services'. (p 39) They draw attention to Lee and Pithers (1980) who point out the problems associated with 'effectively detaching the individual from the social' (p 39) and also Baldwin (1990) who states, 'we must beware of perpetuating services which plan their interventions solely on the individual level' (p 39) The tensions that exist between individual and group aspects within care settings are not actually worked through in any of the literature.

As an unresearched area of the residential experience, the variability of the quality of practice has been brought out in anecdotal reporting. This has also been verified within the writer's own previous personal experience. A lack of a clear conceptual base (discussed briefly within this chapter) may possibly be coupled in some settings with a 'low key' approach to requirements. This, it may be suggested, can render keyworking a meaningless concept/idea within many establishments. Yet armchair theorists, and much of the anecdotal reporting, clearly argues that keyworking can be meaningful in application, and valuable in creating an effective base for individualising the experience of service users within the wider context of residential settings.

This book seeks to establish the nature and context of sound practice through keyworkers. It seeks to explore the themes in practice that may improve keyworker systems and the themes which may be present as inherent weaknesses in formulations of keyworker practice. This book explores the central question: Does keyworking in residential care for older people contribute towards improved individualised care?

4. The structure of the book

This chapter has so far considered the rationale and purpose of the book. Chapter 2 seeks to establish a research agenda (located within that rationale and purpose) from themes found within the literature concerning keyworking. The themes form the basis of initial research questions that were posed. These questions (i) set the context of keyworking within establishments; (ii) concern the overall effect of keyworker systems in residential care for older people; (iii) concern the practice of relationships in keyworker systems; and (iv) concern the practice of decision making and meeting needs in keyworker systems.

Chapter 3 moves on to consider the basis of research methods utilised. The research questions from the previous chapter formed a platform to consider the methodology required to explore the nature of the actual practice of keyworking and the context within which it occurs. The previous research questions were thus placed into two groups: those demanding contextual exploration and those requiring extensive practice exploration. Two stages in the research design, both small scale explorations, were then established: (1) The context and effect of keyworking was considered in a survey questionnaire filled in by managers of establishments with keyworkers; and (2) The nature of the practice of keyworkers in individualising care was considered by case study examination of a small number of individual establishments. This research design combined quantitative and qualitative methodology in order to enable a broader understanding of the nature of keyworking.

Chapter 4 examines findings, from the survey which was conducted as the first stage of the research methodology (as formulated in the previous chapter). These findings denote the context and effect of keyworking. They provide a base from which to conduct research on the practice of keyworking in the next two chapters.

Chapters 5 and 6 thus paint a picture of keyworking practice, firstly in a large statutory establishment, and secondly, in a small private sector establishment. These two establishments were selected from the previously conducted survey. The methodology used here accords with that established in chapter 3 for this stage of the research. The keyworker systems were ones in which particularly important responses to practice requirements had been made. Practice was reported using details given in interviews with keyworkers, supervisors, managers, service users and relatives. The particular strengths and weaknesses of these keyworker systems (in contributing towards improved individualised care) were teased out through the exploration of the themes previously highlighted in the literature search in chapter two. The overall impression in both establishments was a variability in the nature and quality of practice on many of the dimensions explored.

Arising out of this discussion and a consideration of findings relating to the context of keyworking (as previously discussed in chapter 4) Chapter 7 assessed the implications of differing systems and practices, making recommendations for policy, strategy, organisation and practice. This process was carried out within the broad themes suggested by the previous literature search (chapter 2).

The analysis indicated that keyworking in residential care for older people does contribute towards improved individualised care. Practice is particularly effective when considered within the broader context of group living and the overall work of the staff team. Its effectiveness is, however, dependent upon the calibre of a broad tapestry of systems and structures (in particular those concerning supervision, evaluation and care planning), how these are utilised within keyworker systems and upon the nature of the individual keyworker/ service user relationship. The weakness of the concept lies in the variability of practice and relationships within establishments when minimum standards and requirements are not defined and/or not applied.

Thus in Chapter 2 we now commence the journey that later concludes with these analytical findings. That journey has just been mapped out in this section. Chapter 2 commences the process of formulating an answer to the question: Does keyworking in residential care for older people contribute towards improved individualised care? The book continues with an exploration of the historical and contemporary writings concerning keyworking in residential care.

2 Themes in the context and practice of keyworking

1. Introduction

This chapter seeks to establish a research agenda from themes within the literature concerning keyworking. These themes may then form the basis of research into the nature of the actual practice of keyworking and the context that it occurs within.

As was highlighted in the previous chapter, a keyworker is the person who is responsible for the individual care of service users based upon personalised relationships within the context of the group setting. A lack of clarity concerning what this actually means, and a tension between individualised and group responses to the provision of care, renders this an idea that is open to many mixed interpretations each differentially affecting the basis of practice.

In establishing secure foundations for research to answer the question: Does keyworking in residential care for older people contribute towards improved individualised care? this chapter focuses upon broad themes arising out of the historical and the contemporary writings concerning keyworking. These themes will then enable an overall agenda to be set for the research. In order to make sense of a disparate and largely unanalytical literature base, the themes will avoid a partial focus upon divergent individual aspects of the wide diversity of keyworker practice. They will focus upon common threads linking practice and how these interrelate into a general picture of the issues involved. They will enable an overall sense of these issues to be obtained, and how they may contribute to a secure and firm foundation for research into keyworking as a methodology for individualising care.

2. Historical survey: varieties of keyworking

Over a period of eighteen years since keyworking practice commenced post 1976 considerable shifts have thus occurred in the nature of the role of keyworkers. There has been a wide diversity of practice. There has not been a unified or analytic view of the concept. In order to put the themes (that are to be explored below) into context, it is necessary to explore briefly the historical development of keyworking and the different types of keyworking that have applied in settings other than residential care.

In the 1960s and generally up to circa 1975 individual workers in children's homes often paired up with their opposite numbers in fieldwork in order to enable informed decisions about the children in their care (Younghusband 1978). This appears to have formed the basis for policy initiatives formulated by working parties meeting in 1976 to enable named individuals to progress decision making across organisational boundaries existing between fieldwork and residential care. RCA/BASW (1976, 347) defined a keyworker as 'the person having full responsibility for the service user received into residential care and for decisions relating to the case.' They elaborate this as covering all stages (pre-admission, admission and rehabilitation) and spanning all the settings involved. The keyworker's primary focus was upon decision making and co-ordination through different stages of care (pre-admission, admission and rehabilitation).

This was followed (during the period circa 1976-1979) by practitioners and managers endeavouring to put these policies into practice. Difficulties encountered concerned who did what, how they did it and to whom were they accountable. (Rodway 1979; and Davis 1978). During the period circa 1980-1984, it became generally acknowledged that formal boundary spanning roles in keyworking in residential care was not practical, but that keyworking offered a new way of providing care through individual personal relationships, particularly within residential settings (Hogan 1988; RCA 1984; Burningham 1983). Thus there developed (during the period circa 1984 to 1989) a fuller recognition of the potential of providing residential care through individualised relationships within an internal keyworker role. Principles of practice were established (Meteyard 1986; Mallinson 1987; Mallinson and Citarella 1990). It is this form of keyworking that is debated in this book.

The relatively clear sense of focus in residential care may be contrasted with keyworking in other settings. A proliferation of different keyworker types based upon co-ordination of planning and /or direct care provision occurred circa the early 1980's. These covered all sorts of settings each of which formed differing kinds of systems. There were only a few common elements to these. (NISW 1982; SCA/BASW 1987). The spectrum of roles focused on the one hand upon relationships, and at the other end of the spectrum upon co-ordination. (NISW 1982; SCA/BASW 1987; Dubois, Mockler and Mockler 1984).

The coordinating role of a named individual offered a means to cut through the problems of multi-disciplinary work. A named individual provided a single door for the service user to knock on. (SCA/BASW 1987; Riordan, Bramhall and Backhouse 1988; Glendinning 1986; Challis, Darton, Johnson and Stone 1988). Keyworkers were also used as a means to provide 'named persons' coordinating work in specific statutory situations. Keyworking in child abuse investigations is of particular note here. (DHSS 1976; and BASW 1985). Similarly the keyworker as a named individual responsible for the purchasing activities of case/care management in community care occurred circa the early 1990s. (Beardshaw and Towell 1990; Bulmer 1987; Dant et al 1989; Mallinson 1989a; Mallinson and Kelly 1990).

According to SCA/BASW (1987), within residential care establishments, keyworker systems address the purpose of individualisation of care focusing primarily upon decision making to meet needs through direct close intimate continuing relationships. Keyworking within child abuse teams and community mental handicap teams enable clarity of responsibility and decision – making in care planning processes that primarily involve keyworkers in much less intimate co-ordination roles enabling multi – disciplinary contact.

Keyworking in residential care thus primarily concerns the provision of individualised care through relationships. Milestones in the development of principles for keyworking within residential care have been:

- Burningham (1983) highlighted relationships in relation to decision making;
- Fewster (1979) analysed treatment and therapy based upon keyworker roles within a team approach;
- Meteyard (1986?) suggested how roles may be negotiated in relation to personalised care and organisational issues;
- Fletcher (1985) explored frameworks to tackle social, emotional and physical health through individualisation of care;
- Taylor (1985) and Howe (1990) examined personal responsibility in the assessment and management of risk.

These principles have now evolved in the 1990s into practice that is generally conducted within keyworker systems that work to the definition of keyworking that is utilised in this book: Keyworking in residential care for older people is 'a system for providing individualised social care through named persons. A keyworker is the person who has responsibility and accountability for the care of the service user and for decisions relating to their situation.' (SCA, 1991).

Much of the historical debates that concern (for example) spanning boundaries between residential care and fieldwork, and continuity of experience between sectors no longer apply in the ways that they are framed within the literature.

Themes in current practice form the basis of the way actions undertaken by keyworkers are defined and the quality (or otherwise) of the resulting outcomes. The themes that affect current practice may be placed under the two broad headings of relationships within residential care and decision making/meeting needs.

3.1 Themes in current keyworking practice: (a) relationships

In considering an overview of themes concerning relationships in keyworker practice in residential care for older people it is useful to first examine general explorations by Burningham (1983) and Rodway (1981). The broader pattern of relationships is also examined in the literature (Hopkins et al. 1984)

Burningham (1983) saw the keyworker's task as one of helping residents to organise and enjoy their lives, to offer both care and companionship on an individual and continuous basis just as a close friend or relative might do since the act of doing something together builds up relationships. Rodway (1981) continues this theme by considering 'the special relationship' between the worker and service user.

Rodway also considers group interaction as central to keyworking. This may be linked with the view of Hopkins et al. (1984) who state that the role of the keyworker is shaped not only by the perceptions of the keyworker but by the expectations of others. The keyworker is part of the life space of the service user. The therapeutic role, in rebuilding relationships or constructing new opportunities, is clearly mentioned here. Job enrichment in the introduction of keyworker systems is a positive move, helping to enable keyworkers to give service users a sense of belonging. Keyworkers need the attributes of natural warmth, empathy and genuineness in their approach to others.

All these papers provide a basis for consideration of meaning and personal relevance in interactions and relationships between keyworkers and service users within arrangements for group living. Sharing of interests between keyworkers and service users is one particular dimension of this. A range of factors appears to also affect the nature of the individual professional relationship between keyworkers and service users. These are suggested in the literature to be initiated within a process of matching when initial allocations of work are made.

Factors often considered here in this process include the purpose of the placement (eg. needs, problems, length of assistance, the care plan and possible restoration to independent living); The previous and current experience of the client and of the worker (age, sex, cultural and religious factors, skills, experience and training, workload and availability, relationships with other professionals and the client). RCA (1976, 1978 and 1983) and Mallinson and Citarella (1990). Hogan (1988) suggests the integration of matching and task definition. Where co-working is practised, Mallinson and Best (1987) suggest client choice is increased in relation to relationships.

Themes that involve relationships within current practice in keyworking in residential care for older people may thus be classified into those concerning:

- Group living (particularly in relation to small groups),
- Sharing of interests between keyworkers and service users,
- Matching/Allocation of service users to keyworkers, and
- Co-keyworking.

Each of these is now examined in detail in turn.

1. Group living

Group living sets the context for keyworking given the issues we have raised regarding the tension between individualising care and the group experience. Historically (RCA/BASW 1976) sought to improve standards of practice in relation to the continuity of experience for service users. To some extent part of this was the group living experience involved. This and most of the literature that sought to establish codified principles of practice and tools for practice development (eg. RCA <1976> <1983>) concentrates, however, upon individualised care planning, implementation, monitoring progress, reviews, records and maintaining individual relationships rather than the overall small group experience.

In examining developments sequentially it appears that other countries also grappled with issues of individualisation in residential care at this time. For example, in the context of human relationships of a USA setting which promoted a total treatment milieu for mentally ill people, Bettelheim (1974) comments upon how patients and members of staff create their own joint commitments to fulfil special and personalised individual needs based upon deep and sensitive dyadic relationships within the context of small group living.

Back in the UK Bromley (1977) discussed the 'prime care agent' as the person responsible for enabling key decisions eg. entry to residential care. It was maintained that the 'quality of interaction' which also implied small living groups was the most significant factor in effectiveness. Mallinson (1989b); and Mallinson and Best (1987) examine networks of relationships, in relation to decision making and care planning.

Burningham (1983) explored relationships in terms of companionship, and 'doing things together' in small groups. In Taylor (1985) keyworkers had a primary role in a particular establishment for the delivery of individualised care; each keyworker was responsible for service users within the overall group living arrangement.

SCA (1988) attempted to provide a formula locating keyworking firmly within the wider framework for the delivery of care. Here the principles of the management of keyworking systems are also explored in detail. The caring in homes initiative practice guide on communication (SCA, 1993c) gives aspects of keyworker systems that may be developed to enable increased communication throughout residential practice including commonality of experience between residents and keyworkers.

The problem of balancing individual and collective interests appears not to have been fully addressed in the literature. The allocation of an individual keyworker implies individualised systems of care, yet users and keyworkers 'are part of a wider group within residential establishments.' (Elkan and Kelly, 1991 p 39) Thus a tension of balancing individual choice against the interests of the wider residential community appears to exist. The tension between small group living and the establishment as a whole is also part of this.

Nonetheless, a small number of positive evaluative studies exist that point to positive results from keyworker systems, in the context of the small group experience. For example DHSS study (1979) in the course of examining wider aspects of quality in residential care found that where each staff member had a special responsibility for a group of service users, there was evidence that they knew the users better and that pressure on staff was less. (see Lishman, 1982 p 144).

A single question that may fruitfully be raised in this book in relation to the context of actual practice, is therefore:

> What is the relationship between keyworking and small group living?

Issues that might be usefully explored in relation to practice within this theme are: how individual needs are met within the group context, the commonality of experience of residents in individualising care within a group context and the balance of individual choice and the interests of the wider residential community.

Subsidiary questions that would also set the specific context of keyworking relative to the group experience would also include:

> How many service users are allocated to each keyworker?

> What staffing arrangements are made in keyworker systems?

In addition, bearing in mind the confusion regarding the terminology utilised for named individuals providing individualised care within living groups (illustrated within the preceding discussion where prime care agent is used instead of the title of keyworker, and also linkworkers as highlighted in the discussion below) it is useful to ask the contextual question:

What terms are used for keyworkers or equivalent roles?

2. Sharing of interests between keyworkers and service users

Burningham (1983) explored relationships between keyworkers and service users, in terms of companionship, and 'doing things together'. Similarly, in residential care for adolescents Fewster (1979) comments upon an abandonment of a houseparent system at an establishment located in Canada and its replacement with the keyworker concept whereby 'each child related to one special staff member with whom he could become involved'. (p 240) In Fletcher (1985) keyworking enables the special needs of service users to be worked with. Tossell and Webb (1986) describe the role as 'developing a special trusting relationship that ensures that the child benefits from a warm concern that encourages confidential communication of needs and assists the child to develop the confidence to take an interest in a determine his future.' (p 197)

The Caring in Homes Initiative practice guide on communication (SCA, 1993c) give aspects of keyworker systems that may be developed to enable amongst other things, commonality of experience between residents and keyworkers.

Given the ambiguity of the literature, ie whether relationships are based upon sharing the companionship and friendship of mutual interests, or based entirely upon a professional role, it will be useful to ask the question in this research: What is the nature of the keyworker/ service user relationship?

3. Matching/allocation of service users to keyworkers

RCA/BASW (1976) set out a rudimentary typology of factors that the working party felt should be taken into account in choosing a keyworker. This particular approach to allocation was further developed in later literature (eg. RCA 1983) that sought to establish codified principles for practice development. Factors considered here included the purpose of the placement (eg. needs, problems, length of assistance, the care plan and possible restoration to independent living); The previous and current experience of the client and of the worker (age, sex, cultural and religious factors, skills, experience and training, workload and availability, relationships with other professionals and the client).

Following Douglas and Payne (1983), Hogan (1988) suggested that residents and keyworkers should be 'matched' according to the task in hand based upon an analysis of the proposed role.

Mallinson and Citarella (1990) further define and debate principles of practice in matching individual keyworkers and service users. These largely follow RCA/BASW (1976) and RCA (1983). Factors of gender and race are particularly explored in relation to feelings and emotions of service users and ways of proceeding in the process of matching outlined.

All these papers consist of theoretical approaches that have not been tested by research. Thus for this book two questions may be posed:

> How are keyworkers matched to service users?
>
> What are the criteria and methods used?

4. Co-keyworking

Two workers acting jointly 'co-keyworking' in residential care is discussed in Mallinson and Best (1987). This is also examined in joint working between residential social workers and teachers in special education (Mallinson, 1989b). Both these works are the only ones that examine co-working by keyworkers. They do so in relation to the network of relationships, in the process of decision making and care planning. These are theoretical works only. Thus in examining keyworker systems and the basis of working, two questions should be raised:

> How widespread is the practice of co-keyworking?
>
> How does co-keyworking operate?

3.2 Themes in current keyworking practice: (b) decision making in meeting needs

Relationships appear to form a basic aspect of keyworking that concern decision making in meeting needs. In considering an overview of themes concerning decision making in keyworker practice in residential care for older people, it is useful to first consider the question of who makes the rules within relationships and within daily living. In doing this, Burningham (1983) flags up the importance of ethos in relation to roles taken by keyworkers and planning care undertaken by them.

Ward (1978, p1) suggests that a keyworker system offers: 'a framework for deciding and implementing a programme of care *plus goal directed activity* specific to each resident . . . the keyworker's task is to ensure that a viable plan of action exists, that the resident is included at all stages of the plan and that opportunities are provided for implementing the agreed activities within a defined time scale, he is responsible for day to day decision making and is accountable to the case conference team.' Sackville (1979) highlighted the process of keyworking in relation to care planning: 'ensuring that an individual care plan is evolved . . . updating . . . implementing . . . monitoring progress . . . reviews . . . .' Mallinson (1989a) gave a framework for such a care planning and explored some principles involved.

The keyworker's responsibility for decision making in care planning was further outlined by Pragnell (1983) in terms of accountable structures and requirements. Responsibility for the 'evolution' and implementation of the care plan, monitoring progress and calling reviews are part of the role and processes envisaged. Elliott (1978) places this within the context of overall processes of change and levels of working in an establishment. Mallinson (1989a) is specific in terms of requirements for individual care planning in the context of the overall aims and philosophy of the establishment as a whole. Howe (1990) briefly mentions the responsibility of 'linkworkers' in managing risk.

Themes that involve decision making and meeting needs within current practice in keyworking in residential care for older people may thus be classified into those concerning:

- Tasks undertaken by keyworkers,
- Networking by keyworkers,
- Care planning activities undertaken by keyworkers, and
- Decision making in daily living.

Each of these is now examined in detail, in turn.

1. Tasks undertaken by keyworkers

The literature establishes the nature of the role of keyworkers within which the tasks they undertake are founded. These set a major basis of the context of keyworker practice. Ward (1978) for example, highlighted the keyworker as the person responsible for 'deciding, and implementing a programme of care plus goal – directed activity specific to each resident'. RCA (1983) defined the role of keyworker in relation to individualised care planning, implementation, monitoring progress, reviews, records and maintaining relationships Douglas and Payne (1987) suggested that 'each (residential or day care) unit tends to develop its own prescription of duties for its keyworkers'.

Meteyard (1986?) suggests how roles and tasks for individualisation may be developed and agreed with those involved. Fulcher and Ainsworth (1985) describe keyworker responsibilities in group care for children, where a direct care worker co-ordinates all aspects of care and treatment for a particular child. 'The primary task of a keyworker is to be a special person in the eyes of the child and to be responsible for liaison with others on behalf of that child. As the person who has (the) most information about the child and his situation, she/he will be responsible for overall plans and will need to have authority to make decisions.' (p 230) Activities carried out by the keyworker '. . . might include planning care and treatment . . . report writing, liaison concerning job finding or school attendance, formal counselling sessions, working with the family and so on'. (p 101-102)

Domoney and Halves (1989) provide a directory of practice examples in residential care for elderly people. The focus of the task concerns involvement of care staff (Bexley), review (Coventry, Dorset, Wakefield, Surrey, & Kingston on Thames), admissions (Cumbria, Surrey, & Fife), enabling independence (East Sussex, Surrey, & North Tyneside), care planning (Greenwich) and assessment (a private establishment in Bolton).

SCA in their research link keyworking and other trends in tasks undertaken by care assistants. (SCA 1992a) suggests that, 'There appears to have been a . . . shift in emphasis in the daily work of many care assistants, 'to act as keyworker, to be involved in assessment, attend reviews, (and) complete reports'. The care assistants . . . have not argued against these trends . . . (although their job is still) . . . about providing personal care and the domestic labour which supports it.'

Following Cambridge (1992) and Dant and Gearing (1990) keyworkers in residential care will assume some direct care support for individual service users. They have the potential to enable service user's day to day needs to be monitored and support to be provided. The detailed knowledge of service users that is necessary for planning may be gained through such daily contact. Keyworkers will therefore (in addition to their direct caring role) liaise closely with decision makers, feeding information directly into IPP or case reviews, or indirectly via other workers such as case/care managers.

With the notable exception of the SCA study (SCA, 1992a) all these discussions of the role and the tasks undertaken by keyworkers are entirely prescriptions for practice. Thus, in this book two questions should be posed:

> What tasks are undertaken by keyworkers and what is the order of their importance?
>
> What are the limitations of the role of the keyworker?

2. Networking by keyworkers

Networking was an early issue in embryonic keyworking practice. Younghusband (1978) states that a pattern in residential care for children 'emerged by degrees (which) made caseworkers (in residential settings responsible for particular residents and their families – often before admission – in co-operation with resident staff as well as for after care . . . .' (Vol. 2, p 178). Ward (1978) however discussed the subsequent underplaying of the emergent ideal of a keyworker as the person who was responsible for the 'progress through' (pre-admission, admission, and later, discharge and after care) of a service user in relation to relationships within the residential experience.

Following Cambridge (1992) and Dant and Gearing (1990) keyworkers in residential care now (in addition to their direct caring role) need to liaise closely with decision makers, feeding information directly into IPP or case reviews, or indirectly via other workers such as case/care managers.

In the context of other questions concerning meeting needs, the question may thus be raised in this book:

> With which other professionals do keyworkers have regular contact?

3. Care planning activities

Historically the 'keyworker' as 'the person having full responsibility for the service user received into residential care' was to be responsible for 'decisions relating to the case.' (RCA/BASW 1976). Ward (1978) discussed the subsequent underplaying of the ideal of a keyworker as the person who was responsible for the 'progress through' (pre-admission, admission, and later, discharge and after care) of a service user in relation to relationships within the residential experience. She highlighted the keyworker as the person responsible for 'deciding, and implementing a programme of care plus goal – directed activity specific to each resident'. The principle of planning and progressing/ coordinating care was clearly delineated. This formed the basis for later work (eg. RCA 1983) where the foundations of subsequent methodology in care planning may be found.

The view that the role of keyworker is central in care planning processes occurs throughout the literature. For example, RCA 1976 and 1983 sought to define the role of keyworker in relation to individualised care planning, implementation, monitoring progress, reviews, records and maintaining relationships. Howe (1990) suggests that 'linkworkers' take personal responsibility for the care of one particular child and play a key role in the assessment and management of risk. Fletcher (1985) uses keyworking as a framework to tackle issues such as the individual service user's social, emotional and physical health. Fulcher and Ainsworth (1985) describe keyworker responsibilities in group care for children, where a direct care worker co-ordinates all aspects of care and treatment for a particular child. 'The primary task of a keyworker is to be a special person in the eyes of the child and to be responsible for liaison with others on behalf of that child. As the person who has (the) most information about the child and his situation, she/he will be responsible for overall plans and will need to have authority to make decisions.' (p 230) Activities carried out by the keyworker '. . . might include planning care and treatment . . . , report writing, liaison concerning job finding or school attendance, formal counselling sessions, working with the family and so on' (p 101-102). The authors suggest that an action plan should describe how the keyworker would carry out these tasks and the plan should be incorporated as a formal feature of the service (p 101).

Given the fact that all these works are again prescriptive theorising, and that no direct research evidence exists regarding care planning in keyworker systems, nor how needs are met, the question may now be asked:

How are the needs of service users met within keyworker systems?

4. Decision making in daily living

The initial RCA/BASW (1976) document explored basic principles of accountability in decision – making, and cooperative approaches. Following this, Davis (1978) expressed the organisational problems and constraints that had become significant given ambiguities in the keyworker proposals. He specifically mentions 'the shadow of accountability . . . (and) . . . divided loyalties' in the context of confidentiality, communication, and power in/ the power of relationships. In identifying the structural problem of an employee who is expected to be accountable to both service user and manager, Davis also notes with concern that the keyworker may be incorporated into a 'spurious consensus' with other professional colleagues at the expense of the weakest party – the service user. Davis however quoted situations where keyworkers had developed relationships with service users of such quality that they became totally available and involved as advocates for service user's rights and champions in individualised development. Davis (1978) highlighted a basic issue, that as a decision maker, a keyworker could only be as good as other workers and the system would allow.

Fulcher and Ainsworth (1985) link decision making in daily living with care planning. They describe keyworker responsibilities in group care for children, where a direct care worker co-ordinates all aspects of care and treatment for a particular child. 'The primary task of a keyworker is to be a special person in the eyes of the child and to be responsible for liaison with others on behalf of that child. As the person who has (the) most information about the child and his situation, she/he will be responsible for overall plans and will need to have authority to make decisions' (p 230). Activities carried out by the keyworker '. . . might include planning care and treatment . . . , report writing, liaison concerning job finding or school attendance, formal counselling sessions, working with the family and so on' (p 101-102).

SCA (1988) attempted to provide a formula locating keyworking firmly within the wider framework for the delivery of care. Here the principles of the management of keyworking systems are also explored in detail. Thus keyworking forms part of a wider structure within which to implement principles, and objectives.

SCA (1992b) states that keyworking in residential care for older people provides a structure. Responsibility, accountability and decision-making appear to be issues here. SCA also state 'A keyworker system can improve communication and continuity of care' (p 19). It appears from this document that keyworking provides a basis for the implementation of sound principles of individualised care. Similarly, in discussing ways of enabling good practice by creating black perspectives in residential care, Jones et al. (1992) state that keyworker systems are valuable since they provide service users with a sense of continuity. They also state that they should not occur in isolation from interaction with staff, 'as the effects of staff sickness and annual leave have to be taken into account of, and planned for accordingly' (p 32).

The caring in homes initiative practice guide on communication (SCA, 1993c) give aspects of keyworker systems that may be developed to enable increased communication: commonality of experience between residents and keyworkers, matching, guidelines that take into account the concerns of keyworkers and residents, availability of staff, relationships of trust and friendship, and the support of managers.

Arising out of these issues in the literature, the single most important question in this area that it is appropriate to ask in this study would appear to be:

What is the authority, responsibility and accountability of keyworkers?

4. The overall effect of keyworker systems

Kelly and Harris (1991) have commented upon the broad tapestry of principles and the diversity of provision that emerged in keyworking in residential care. They clearly state that which ever variant is adopted by managers for particular settings, 'the principle of having a designated member of staff particularly responsible for the needs of a service user or a small group of service users is accepted as good practice.' They continue by stating that 'keyworking had probably been the single most influential idea in social care.'

A small number of positive evaluative studies exist that point to positive results from keyworker systems. These particularly focus upon the area of decision making and daily living. A DHSS study (1979) in the course of examining wider aspects of quality in residential care found that where each staff member had a special responsibility for a group of service users, there was evidence that they knew the users better and that pressure on staff was less (see Lishman, 1982 p 144). A more recent research study again concerning wider questions within care services for older people (Counsel and Care, 1992) contained a single short paragraph advocating a greater use of keyworkers. They found in London that 49% of all older people who were general service users would wish to have one member of staff working closely with them as an individual '. . . and 23% expected it . . . . (17%) of those now in (private and voluntary) homes actually had a keyworker.'

It may be suggested that the accumulation of practice wisdom concerning keyworking in residential care has been patchy, yet the evidence in the Wagner report (NISW, 1988, Vol. 1, page 197) had '. . . a great many favourable references to the keyworker concept.' The evidence states that it was seen by some as '. . . the most significant development in residential care for all client groups' and its 'promising development owed as much to improving the work satisfaction and contribution of staff as . . . to ensuring that resident's needs are met effectively'.

In the context of this literature review as a whole in setting the research agenda, it is thus pertinent to ask a small number of questions evaluating keyworker systems as a whole. These may be:

> What is the effect of keyworker systems upon areas such as individualised care, and relationships?
>
> Do keyworker systems result in any clarification of the residential task?

5. Conclusions: a research agenda

Teasing out the themes concerning the effect of individualised care through keyworking isolates areas pertinent to research. Investigation of these themes should provide information through which to answer that central question: Does keyworking in residential care for older people contribute towards improved individualised care? The areas/themes are now summarised in the form of initial research questions:

Questions that set the context of keyworking within establishments:

> What is the relationship between keyworking and small group living?
>
> What terms are used for keyworkers or equivalent roles?
>
> How many service users are allocated to each keyworker?
>
> What staffing arrangements are made in keyworker systems?
>
> What tasks are undertaken by keyworkers and what is the order of their importance?

With which other professionals do keyworkers have regular contact?

How are keyworkers matched to service users? What are the criteria and methods used?

How widespread is the practice of co-keyworking? How does co-keyworking operate?

Questions concerning the overall effect of keyworker systems in residential care for older people:

What is the effect of keyworker systems upon areas such as individualised care, and relationships?

Do keyworker systems result in any clarification of the residential task?

Questions concerning the practice of relationships in keyworker systems:

What is the nature of the keyworker service user relationship?

Questions concerning the practice of decision making and meeting needs in keyworker systems:

What are the limitations of the role of the keyworker?

How are the needs of service users met within keyworker systems?

What is the authority, responsibility and accountability of keyworkers?

These questions arising out of the themes in the literature search form an agenda for the research undertaken to explore the context and practice of keyworking in residential care for older people in this book. The methodology upon which that research was to be conducted and the framework involved forms the subject of the next chapter.

3 Research methods

1. Introduction

The previous chapter indicated the complex interrelationships of factors around themes involved in individualised care by keyworkers. The questions arising from these themes formed a starting point in considering research methodology. The questions were felt to fall into two groups: those demanding contextual exploration and those requiring extensive practice exploration.

Two stages in the research design, both small scale explorations, were thus considered:

(1) The context and effect of keyworking was established by a survey questionnaire filled in by managers of establishments with keyworkers (forming a sub-part of a much broader questionnaire administered as a census of all establishments for older people within a defined geographical area). The survey explored general aspects of keyworking such as the tasks keyworkers undertake, the process of matching, the extent and basis of co-keyworking, and the wider context of staffing and living arrangements.

(2) The nature of the practice of keyworkers in individualising care was established by case study examination of a small number of individual establishments. The significance and meaning of providing individualised care through keyworking for that establishment, the service users and staff was examined. Here interviews with managers, staff, service users and relatives got to grips with practice, processes and role of keyworkers. The interviews attempted to assess how service users' views of requirements, processes and outcomes and their meaning for everyday living were translated into practice requirements.

The use of these two stages reflect dual traditions in social research. The combining of quantitative and qualitative methodology according to Bryman (1988) enables a broader understanding of different aspects of the phenomenon in question. The quantitative methodology of stage one allowed the context to be set for the qualitative case studies explored in stage two. This dual exploration of the issues permitted the defining and exploration of themes in greater depth. The logic of this is discussed in Webb et al (1966). The specific nature of the themes explored within the case studies were grounded from within the contextual findings of the survey.

2. Stage one: survey questionnaire

Themes and research questions

The themes in the literature search suggested general contextual questions for research that would be amenable to exploration through a questionnaire:

What terms are used for keyworkers or equivalent roles?

Is there a relationship between keyworkers and small living groups?

How many service users are allocated to each keyworker?

What staffing arrangements are made in keyworker systems?

What tasks are undertaken by keyworkers and what is the order of their importance?

With which other professionals do keyworkers have regular contact?

How are keyworkers matched to service users? What are the criteria and methods used?

How widespread is the practice of co-keyworking? How does co-keyworking operate?

What is the effect of keyworker systems upon areas such as individualised care, and relationships?

Do keyworker systems result in any clarification of the residential task?

These questions were ones where considerable variation may occur between different establishments. As contextual questions and questions considering general aspects of practice, the questionnaire method was felt to be the most appropriate to utilise in order to establish common threads throughout keyworker systems and the degree of variation that may exist between systems.

From these research questions exploring the context of keyworking, the survey of keyworking establishments conducted within the broader census questionnaire was constructed.

The nature of the census

The postal census of all residential care establishments for older people (ie. all those in the statutory, voluntary and private sectors) within a defined geographical area was undertaken by the author as part of a wider study. Only aspects of the census that are relevant to keyworking are discussed within this book.

The census took place within the entire territory of the following West Midlands Metropolitan District Councils: Birmingham, Dudley, Sandwell, Walsall and Wolverhampton. The frame for the census was complied from local authority registration and inspection records. It may be said to be fully comprehensive: given the legal requirement to register. Any private or voluntary sector establishment not so registered would be operating illegally. For the statutory sector information was obtained from the providing authority owning all the establishments.

A census of all establishments in a defined (narrow) geographical area contrasts with (for example) a 10% national survey. A national survey was not possible at the time because of the absence of a national database to give information from which an adequate sample frame could be constructed. Practical considerations determined a West Midlands location for the census. Local knowledge was available to the author that indicated broadly the likely composition of the census frame. In encapsulating an entire geographical area the census/survey was designed to be fairly comprehensive. The assumption was made that keyworker systems in this location would reflect issues that pertained to other geographical areas, although generalisations beyond the West Midlands should be made with caution. For example, no comparative information in relation to other parts of the country was available concerning individual needs of service users. Results may thus be seen as valid rather than as necessarily having a wider reliability.

The wording of the census questionnaire was formulated utilising the guiding principles outlined by Moser and Kalton (1971). The approach adopted was that the accompanying letter was brief but gave essential information (on the purpose, and what is to be done with the information); the questionnaire is carefully and clearly laid out with clear instructions; and questions are simple and clear. The questionnaire was 'tested' with several colleagues who would (as officers in charge) be in receipt of the final version. Subsequent minor modifications were then made as a result of these discussions.

The questionnaire was sent to the Manager or Officer in Charge of each establishment as the normal contact point for receipt of mail. The response is therefore conducted from the perspective of the management of the establishment and does not necessarily directly reflect the views of keyworkers or service users. A covering letter and a stamped addressed envelope was sent with the questionnaire.

The questionnaire was constructed in two parts. The first part (relating to the study outwith this book) concerned systems and structures other than keyworking. The second part of the questionnaire was filled in only by those establishments that had keyworkers. From this survey within the census, the data on keyworker systems explored in this book was obtained.

Census/survey: size and response rate

368 Residential establishments for older people existed in the area of the census. The overall census response rate was 102 questionnaires returned (27.27%). This is just above the minimum tolerance level for postal surveys suggested in Moser and Kalton (1971). This low level of response may have resulted from the complexity and extent of answers required. The figure of 27.27% was achieved after a second letter was sent soliciting further responses.

There does not appear to be a strictly comparable methodology utilised in other recent similar research. Thus it is not possible to make comparisons of the response rate in order to assist in the task of reaching a judgement about the reliability of these results. Many methods in analogous research utilise interviews (rather than postal questionnaires). For example, interviews negotiated in homes (Phillips, Vincent and Blacksell, 1989), or interviews following through changes in circumstances of service users (Counsel and Care, 1992). Other studies have used direct collaboration through the line management of local authorities (Booth, 1985). Studies that have utilised postal surveys like Willcocks, Peace and Kellaher (1987) have gone initially through local authority line management. Willcocks et al's particular response rate is not actually recorded.

The composition of keyworking establishments in the survey and its relationship to the main census frame is given below in Table 5.1.

It may be seen from this table that in the proportion of survey responses concerning keyworking are skewed to the statutory sector. This may of course, be simply because there are more statutory establishments with keyworkers. A greater proportion of establishments with keyworkers also replied to the census questionnaire.

Table 3.1:
Census response rate/composition by sector, and composition of survey of establishments with keyworkers

	Voluntary Sector	Private Sector	Statutory Sector	Total
Census				
Questionnaires sent	26	250	92	368
	(7%)	(68%)	(25%)	(100%)
Questionnaires returned	12	53	37	102
(% of returns by Sector)	(46%)	(21%)	(40%)	(100%)
Survey of establishments with keyworkers	6	17	35	58
(% of census returns)	(6%)	(17%)	(35%)	(57%)
(% of survey)	(10%)	(29%)	(60%)	(100%)

The only research that addresses the proportion of service users with keyworkers in residential care for older people that the composition of the survey frame may be compared with (Counsel and Care, 1992) puts the overall figure in a sample of inner and outer London Boroughs at 17%. This related only to the private and voluntary sectors. The comparable figure in the census returns for those sectors would be 35%.

Data analysis

Where appropriate with the small amount of quantitative data relating to keyworking, statistical significance was imputed. The tests used were chi square and the standard error of the difference between means. The standard measures of $p=<0.01$ or $p=<0.05$ were used. Thus these results would be expected to have occurred by chance in only 1 or 5 respectively of every 100 analyses.

Qualitative data obtained from open ended survey questions (such as factors in matching keyworkers and service users) were grouped according to the most logical categorisation suggested by the material. In all cases here the wording in the analysis is faithful to that given by the respondents.

Differences between size of establishments were also grouped according to the most logical categorisation suggested within the material. Small establishments were defined as those of up to 30 service users. Large establishments have been defined as those with 31 or more service users.

Limitations of the survey results

Keyworking is usually a formalised system, yet it would appear that in many establishments practice is carried out as 'keyworking' yet the establishment do not call it by any such technical term. Correspondingly it is not known how many of the establishments in this research with 'keyworkers' are formalising (for the purposes of filling in the survey questionnaire) the informalised. Thus definitive numbers of establishments operating with Keyworker, and therefore the scope of findings in this book, may (around the margins) be open to interpretation.

3. Stage two: interviews in two establishments

Themes and research questions

Stage two of the research moved from the broad context of the survey into case study explorations of the practice of individualised care by keyworkers in two specific residential establishments. Particular questions relating to keyworker practice were suggested by the themes presented in the literature search:

> How are the needs of service users met within keyworker systems?
>
> What are the limitations of the role of the keyworker?
>
> What is the authority, responsibility and accountability of keyworkers?
>
> What is the nature of the keyworker service user relationship?

The quantitative methodology of stage one had allowed the context to be set for these questions. The themes already explored within the survey now provided a grounding for a specific in-depth exploration of the nature and effect of keyworker systems in the two establishments concerned. Thus, the interviews in stage two also incorporated many of the issues previously raised in general terms within the stage one survey. The research questions brought forward in this way from the stage one survey were:

> What is the relationship between keyworking and small group living?
>
> What tasks are undertaken by keyworkers and what is the order of their importance?

With which other professionals do keyworkers have regular contact?

How are keyworkers matched to service users? What are the criteria and methods used?

How widespread is the practice of co-keyworking? How does co-keyworking operate?

What is the effect of keyworker systems upon areas such as individualised care, and relationships?

Do keyworker systems result in any clarification of the residential task?

As all the themes to be considered were ones that required extensive explorations into that practice by individual keyworkers in individual establishments in order to adequately provide answers, they were felt to be particularly amenable to a case study approach. The major factor involved here was the need to assess how the practice of different people (supervisors, managers and keyworkers) interrelated. The meaning of practice for individual service users could also be assessed within the case study. The practice within each establishment involved could be seen in relation to the overall contextual aspects of the study and effect of keyworking discussed in the findings of the previous survey.

Selection of establishments and interviewees

It was decided that two establishments be selected for the second stage of the research, to enable limited comparisons to be made between them. The number of establishments needed to be small so that the intensive work required could be carried out.

Fourteen establishments in the survey indicated their willingness to participate. They were ranked according to suggested quality of their care infrastructure (from the census data) and upon contrasts that could be made between them. One establishment had a co-keyworking scheme; both had small group living provision. One was from the independent sector and one from the statutory sector. One establishment was small (under 30 service users) and one large (30 plus). One (in the ranking of tasks undertaken by keyworkers) had a higher emphasis upon physical care the other upon different functions.

It was clear that there were likely to be differences in perceptions of practice requirements between those involved within the establishments (keyworkers, senior managers, supervisors, service users, and significant others eg. relatives).

In both establishments, a sample of 'keyworkers' (20%) was decided upon to give an adequate picture of keyworker practice in the establishment as a whole. The sample was based upon a balance between those new to the role and those who have carried it out for some time; a balance between full and part time staff; a balance between age, and gender and a balance between dependency of service users matched to the particular keyworkers. The keyworkers were all from differing small living groups. The supervisor of each keyworker was also interviewed.

An initial interview was also held with the officer in charge: to agree the basis of the research, and the interview schedule; explore issues of confidentiality and research ethics; to obtain views on how, in their opinion, the keyworker system operated; obtain the history of the system; and to explore issues of topical interest to staff and service users.

Interviews with each individual keyworker's manager /supervisor then worked to the set the agenda, by discussing themes: ie relationships, small group living, experience of residents, matching, co-keyworking, tasks carried out, networks, role, authority, responsibility and accountability and how the needs of service users are met. Similar interviews were held with each individual keyworker. Differences in perception between keyworkers and supervisors (if any) were openly discussed. The interview checklist reflecting these areas is given in appendix C.

An interview also took place with one of each of the keyworker's allocated service users. The keyworker asked the service user for their permission to be involved. The interview also considered the set themes of the research. For each service user one significant person of their choice involved in the care/planning/friendship network (field social workers, relatives) was interviewed considering the same agenda.

The large statutory establishment in the research had a sheltered housing complex administered from the establishment. As this did not have a keyworker system, this complex was not included in the analysis. The same establishment, some 3/4 of the way through the research process, became under threat of closure. It is possible that this may have altered responses, although efforts were made to keep distortion to a minimum by expressing neutrality in relation to the future status of the establishment.

Safeguarding the trustworthiness of interview material and its interpretation

Qualitative research methods are often criticised on the grounds of 'subjectivity'. These criticisms concern both the methods used, and the researcher's role in collecting and making interpretations from interviews. Leininger (1985) points out that criteria used to determine the reliability and validity of qualitative research are often the same as those used for quantitative research. This is also the view of Bryman (1988). Leininger and Bryman argue that as the purposes, goals and intent of these two types of research differ, different criteria are therefore required to appraise reliability and validity.

It is argued here that the primary purpose of this part of the research ie. to consider the overall nature of practice from the differing perspectives of service users, relatives, keyworkers and managers is interpretive in its approach. Leininger states that qualitative validity rests upon understanding the phenomena as fully as possible. Thus in relation to this study the exploration of different areas in discussion and in interpretive dialogue was felt to be a more valid approach than, for example, a formal questionnaire method.

An intensive case study approach was adopted in this part of the research to enable an adequate description of keyworking practice in the settings studied. Descriptions of aspects of service user's experience are made arising out of examples of keyworking practice discussed.

The validity of interviews with service users (who could feel intimidated by questions concerning the relationship with their keyworker; or, despite explanations, may not fully understand the purpose of the research; or could exhibit a degree of mental confusion) was worked through as much as possible, by careful selection of users in consultation with a particular keyworker's supervisor. The interviews involved sensitive probing, moving at the service user's own pace. The importance of non-verbal communication was not overlooked. Direct questions on occasions teased out differences. The use of jargon was avoided (eg. 'the member of staff whom you do most things with or make decisions with' was used, rather than the term 'keyworker').

In discussing the relationship between keyworkers and their supervisors, the possibility of hidden agendas was endeavoured to be minimised by differences being aired openly. The selection of particular supervisors and keyworkers was determined in consultation with the officer in charge.

According to Burgess (1982) even 'unstructured' interviews should have a structure, as a framework should be established within which the interview is conducted. Interviews are controlled, in that experiences and attitudes elicited should be relevant to the research problem, and the informant should be encouraged to discuss these problems naturally and freely.

The themes covered by the interviews were structured by a checklist (given in appendix C). Open ended questions (eg. 'What do you feel about xxxxx?' or, 'How do you handle yyyy?') with supplementary questions was part of the style of interviews (as was appropriate to the particular interviewee). Free flowing expression of opinion was permissible. The object was to obtain an impression of the nature and the meaning of practice from the point of view of the person involved. The checklists of themes and the basis of interviews were piloted in a different (third) establishment to test their practicality, reliability and validity.

Methods of data analysis

In order to test this methodology and consider the efficacy of answers, a small series of pilot interviews were conducted in another establishment before the main research was progressed. The quality of the record of these interviews were evaluated with the staff involved.

A record of all interviews was constructed immediately after each session, from notes taken during the interview. In the case of some interviews with service users (many of whom were in a confused state) interviews were not fully comprehensive nor were valid responses able to be recorded.

From the interview record an overall sub record was processed relative to each theme of exploration. This was then condensed into analytical statements and conclusions. These form the basis of the discussion presented within this book. Following Burgess (1982) notes concerning themes explored and topics that could be developed were also included in the main substantive field notes in order to aid subsequent analysis, although these notes were distinguished from the direct responses of the informants.

Limitations of the case study data

The selection of keyworkers and residents was carried out by selection of management and supervisors. Similarly the service user/ family was selected by the keyworker. Neither was a random sample. In some cases it appeared that to a certain extent keyworkers had been briefed by their managers immediately before the interview so as to be clear about their role. Non the less, in many instances the position of the keyworker differed radically from that of their manager and this is reflected in the findings. Service users were said to have been selected according to their potential to 'understand' the issues or who were 'particularly interesting' or were simply the 'most lucid' of the group, any of whom would present problems for any interviewer. Overall the main foci of the selection criteria for keyworkers appears to have been who was 'suitable'.

In discussing process divorced from outcome, managers generally appeared to assume that outcomes were successful if there were structures in place. Outcomes where expressed in the interview record do not appear to get to grips with the central issue: what is the actual nature of a relationship and its context, that it may be construed as successful?

The findings show that the practice of delivery of an individualised service through a named individual will have considerable variations depending upon the ability and the values of that individual in relation to the team and managerial context of the setting. Thus action and the continuity of interaction may have a degree of independence that is determined by the beliefs and ideology of the particular individual interviewed.

The notion of the values and manifest power of the keyworker has not been fully explored in the research. Although some of the interviews tentatively explored this issue, the question whether individualised care is too dependent upon the conduct and values of the particular keyworker involved (and therefore whether this negates elements of the principle that keyworker systems present a sound basis upon which individualised care in residential settings may be delivered) has remained unresolved.

The research considered process entirely as a factor in achieving output. Input-output models of service delivery state structures that link activities to the output of the service, ie. to goal achievement. It may be argued that it is only by developing a consensus on the nature of output that that it is possible to attempt to test the validity of pathways to an output systematically. Priorities may be considered in relation to objectives and the logistics of achieving objectives rather than activities or policies themselves. The pressure in measuring effectiveness has thus historically placed the setting of objectives in areas such as local government at the centre of concern (see for example Audit Commission, 1983 and 1986).

More recently documents in social work have taken the perspective that process is of equal, if not prime importance. Booth et al (1990) found for example that a 'cooling effect' occurred in residential care around the implementation of good practice ideas as one moved away from policy devising in the hierarchy to the operational reality in the caring relationship, thus highlighting the importance of process. This has also been the theme of recent quality initiatives such as the 'Caring in Homes Initiative' (eg. Perring, 1992). Both these views post – dated the research design utilised herein. Both express some of the limitations of the research, as it may be argued that Booth's cooling effect is implicit (but not explicitly examined) in the interview record. For example, in stated goals not actually being attained. The analysis therefore has limitations as it partially parallels Booth's findings but was not structured to take formal cognizance or assessment of these elements.

4. Boundaries of the data

There have been shifts in the value base of the service during the five years it has taken to carry out this study. In particular a move towards greater consumerism has taken place. These shifts are encapsulated in changes in the widespread use of terminology. Thus over the five year period 'client' or 'resident' has changed to 'service user' (or to 'user' for short). For the sake of standardisation, the terms 'service user' and 'user' have been used throughout as the standard form in the review of the literature, research record and analysis except where direct quotes are given. In such cases the terms 'resident' or 'client' has been used/ given as in the original. The interview record in stage two (except when quoting verbatim) takes the form of the researcher's own notes and thus the standard terminology has again been used.

The terminology employed for 'keyworker' within the private sector establishment (that the extensive case study was compiled from) was 'primary carer'. In the case study discussion in chapter six, where a persons actual title is referred to, or verbatim quotes made, the term 'primary carer' has been used; where interpretive statements are made, the term 'keyworker' is employed. This has been carried out to enable both consistency and accuracy.

5. Summary and conclusions

The research design consisted of two linked small scale explorations. The first of these explored the context of keyworking by a survey questionnaire filled in by managers of establishments with keyworkers. This formed subpart of a much broader census. The second examined the nature of keyworker practice through case study examination of two individual establishments. The combining of quantitative and qualitative methodology was formulated to enable a broader understanding of different aspects of keyworking. This dual exploration of the issues permitted the defining and exploration of research themes in greater depth.

Specific research themes were suggested from within the literature for investigation to explore the context and practice of keyworking. Additionally some issues were grounded from within the contextual survey for exploration within practice. Steps were taken to safeguard the trustworthiness of the data obtained.

Having set the methodological basis of this book in this chapter, the next stage is to explore some of the findings of the survey setting the context of practice in keyworker systems. That contextual exploration is the subject of the next chapter.

4 The context and effect of keyworking

1. Introduction

Chapter 3 suggested a number of areas that could usefully be explored in representing the context of keyworking practice. These were:

- the range of terms are used for keyworkers or equivalent roles;
- Is there a relationship between keyworkers and small living groups?
- the number of service users allocated to each keyworker;
- the staffing arrangements made in keyworker systems;
- the tasks undertaken by keyworkers and the order of their importance;
- the range of other professionals with whom keyworkers have regular contact;.
- how keyworkers are matched to service users; and
- the practice of co-keyworking.

In addition an exploration of the effect of keyworker systems was suggested in relation to:

- individualised care,
- relationships, and
- the residential task.

This chapter explores the results of the survey for each of these aspects of the context and effect of keyworking in turn.

2. Terms used for 'keyworkers'

The variability of terminology centres upon 'linkworker' and 'keyworker'. This was alluded to in the literature search. The actual usage in establishments in the survey is represented in Table 4.1.

Table 4.1
Terms used for 'keyworkers'

No. of Establishments	Keyworker	Linkworker	Not specified	Other*	TOTAL
Statutory					
Small	6 (100%)	–	–	–	6
Large	22 (76%)	2 (7%)	4 (15%)	1 (4%)	29
Private					
Small	6 (38%)	–	6 (38%)	4 (25%)	16
Large	1 (50%)	–	–	1 (50%)	2
Voluntary					
Small	3 (60%)	–	1 (20%)	1 (20%)	5
Large	1 (100%)	–	–	–	1
TOTAL	39 (66%)	2 (4%)	11 (19%)	7 (12%)	59

*Care manager (although in this particular establishments no mechanisms for care management are reported!), attached worker, senior care assistant, primary workers, special interest worker, rehabilitation assistant, primary nurse, prime carer.

3. Aspects of staffing and living arrangements

Small group living arrangements and keyworking appear in many cases to exist side by side. Indeed establishments with small group living constituted 34% of those with keyworkers (As opposed to the lesser overall incidence of small group living throughout all establishments of 23%). The higher occurrence of small group living arrangements in establishments with keyworkers was particularly marked in statutory establishments (46%).

In establishments with both keyworkers and small group living the size of groups and the number of groups is significantly different between the statutory and the private sectors. The resulting allocation of the number of service users to keyworkers is also significantly different. These findings illustrate the variability that may occur between different keyworker systems in different sectors and presumably variability in the type or style of individualised care that may thus be available (Table 4.2).

Table 4.2
Relationship of keyworking to small group living

	Statutory Est.	Private Est.
Average size of Groups[a]	9.125	7.5
Average number of Groups[b, d]	3.5	2.25
Average number of service users allocated to a keyworker in small group provision[c, e, f]	3.23	4.5

a Standard error = 0.2 significance of difference of the two means p=>5

b Standard error = 0.435 significance of difference of the two means p=>1

c Standard error = 0.35 significance of difference of the two means p=>1

d It should be noted that it is not necessarily the case that a whole establishment is given over to small group living. In some cases establishments (large or small) may only have one small group as part of wider provision.

e Where (in a particular establishment) a range has been given the midpoint of that range has been taken. Differences were given in many establishments between part time and full time staff, often pro rata.

f See also Table 4.3 below.

The mean number of service users allocated to a keyworker in all establishments in the survey was 4.25. Differences (in the number of service users allocated to a keyworker) between establishments with small group living units and establishments without such units were not found to be statistically significant.

It is also useful to explore data giving information concerning staffing in general. This again is so that the backdrop to individualised care by keyworkers may be assessed.

Table 4.3 indicates that individual keyworkers in the survey had more service users allocated to them in the statutory sector compared to the independent sector. Thus there may again be said to be variations in the style and type of individualised care delivery.

Table 4.3
No. of service users allocated to each keyworker: (p=>1, chi square)

	Number of Establishments		
	Statutory	Private	TOTAL
Up to and inc. 3	8 (24%)	8 (33%)	16 (28%)
4/5	21 (62%)	5 (21%)	26 (45%)
Other	5 (15%)	11 (46%)	16 (28%)
TOTAL Est (100%)	34	24	58

Co-keyworking did not appear to be dependent in the survey upon the profile/ratio of full and part time staff in establishments.

Tables 4.4 and 4.5 illustrate that significant differences existed in the census between staffing ratios in establishments with keyworkers compared with those without. Table 4.4 appears to indicate that these differences may simply be a result of more keyworking establishments in the sample being in the statutory sector (where larger establishments predominate). Differences in the number of hours worked by part time staff are of course concealed within this table. Table 4.5 attempts to provide information on the full time equivalent hours worked by part time staff.

Table 4.4
Numbers of establishments with particular levels of full and part time care staff by sector and incidence of keyworker systems

p = >2.5 (Chi sq)	With Keyworkers		Without K	
	Statutory	Ind.	Ind.	TOTAL
0-10 PT Staff	11 (33%)	7 (37%)	25 (64%)	43 (47%)
10+ PT Staff	22 (67%)	12 (63%)	14 (35%)	48 (53%)
Total no. Est (=100%)	33	19	39	91
p = >5 (Chi sq)	With Keyworkers		Without K	
	Statutory	Ind.	Ind.	TOTAL
0-10 FT Staff	13 (39%)	15 (80%)	22 (55%)	50 (54%)
10+ FTe Staff	20 (61%)	5 (20%)	18 (45%)	43 (46%)
Total no. Est (=100%)	33	20	40	93

Table 4.5
Ratios: users to staff

	Est with keyworkers	Est without keyworkers
Mean no of service Users[a]	32	17
No of Part Time Staff (expressed as Full Time Equivalent) per Full Time Staff member[b, d]	1.5	1.8
No of users per Full Time Equivalent Staff Member[c, d]	1.7	1.4

a Standard error = 1.55 significance of difference of the two means p = >1

b Standard error = 0.26 significance of difference of the two means p = >1

c Standard error = 0.05 significance of difference of the two means p = >1

d It is regretted that with the data obtained (subject as it is to wide bandings of part time hours worked) the figures have a degree of inaccuracy. This is why the figures have only been rounded up or down to one decimal point. The mid – point of each band has been taken in all cases. It has been assumed in calculating full time equivalents from part time staff hours that a full time member of staff works 39 hours. Obtaining information on the definitive hours worked by care staff (as distinct from bandings comprising 0-10/10-20/20-30/30+ hours) would enable precise data on full time/ part time ratios, staff ratios in relation to numbers of service users etc. All that the present data gives is a broad picture.

Differences of race/ gender in the composition of service users between establishments with/without keyworkers were found not to be significant in the survey.

Part time staff working under 20 hours per week are less likely to exist in establishments with keyworker systems. This, it may be suggested is due to a need for continuity in relationships in individualised care. Table 4.5 indicates that in the survey fewer part time staff were employed pro rata in establishments with keyworkers thus enabling more cover to be carried out by a single full time keyworker, based upon individual relationships. It may be suggested that service users' individual needs may be met by keyworking on a more continuing basis than may be facilitated by a more transient staff group. Thus individualised care and continuity of care by keyworkers may be linked conceptually.

The number of service users per full time equivalent staff member in the survey is higher in establishments with keyworkers. This may be a function of economies of scale resulting from the larger size of such establishments. This may equally be a function of more of these establishments being in the statutory sector. The question whether the benefits to relationships in individualised care of greater full time cover by keyworkers is on balance negated by the costs to the quality of care of less favourable staffing ratios was not answered within the data.

4. The tasks of keyworkers

Establishments in the survey were asked to rank the tasks that keyworkers undertook. These are analysed in table 4.6.

Previously, Burningham (1983) had surveyed the tasks of keyworkers in one establishment. These had revolved around helping 'residents organise and enjoy their lives.' Other writers have particularly emphasised assessment (Mallinson, 1989a; and Rodway, 1978 & 1981). Counselling (Ward, 1978), recording and admissions (RCA/BASW, 1976) and advocacy (Davis, 1978; and Rodway, 1978 & 1981). SCA/BASW (1987) suggested amongst a number of illustrative tasks: counselling, recording, and physical care.

It would appear in the survey results discussed here, that whilst physical care takes a primary position in the tasks completed by keyworkers, assessment and advocating needs also takes prominence. The needs of a group care setting (supporting daily living) also figure prominently. It is not clear how priorities within the tension between individual needs and group living are determined as the task of supporting daily living is progressed. The role/task of the keyworker as counsellor also is quite high on the list of priorities, this may reflect the individualised service that keyworkers are able to provide. Recording and admissions (tasks that figured prominently in earlier keyworker literature such as RCA/BASW, 1976) do not appear to have the same primary emphasis in current practice.

As a reflection of the structuring of the role of keyworkers, tasks show how particular emphasis within individualised care may be given. The question of how effective action is in carrying out these tasks and what the effect of that action is on the quality of individualised care is explored in the case studies in stage two of this research (chapters 5 and 6).

Table 4.6
Tasks that were ranked 1-5 out of 1-10

Tasks in order of % number of est. within rank 1-5[a]		Percentage of Establishments Statutory Small	Large	Private	Volunt.	ALL EST.
1	Physical Care	100%	89%	100%	75%	94%
2	Support Daily Living	67%	74%	89%	100%	77%
3A	Assessment	100%	77%	67%	100%	74%
3B	Advocate	100%	72%	78%	100%	74%
5	Counselling	33%	47%	88%	67%	54%
6A	Admissions	67%	44%	33%	33%	34%
6B	Recording	67%	50%	25%	33%	34%
6C	Arranging Activities	–	44%	33%	33%	34%
9	Arrange Outings	33%	16%	25%	–	14%
Number of valid responses[b]		3	18	9	3	34

a Other roles stated: Buying clothes, medical, spiritual needs, buying Christmas and birthday presents, medical, liaison with relatives, diet, and 'sitting and listening to resident's joys and worries etc.'

b Many questionnaires were filled in without ranking, rendering their data of little use (particularly as in most of these cases all categories were ticked).

5. Networks with other professionals

There appeared in the survey to be a wide range of networks that keyworkers link into 91% of all keyworkers had direct contact with general practitioners, 53% with field social workers, 81% with district nurses, 74% with chiropodists and 79% with religious leaders. More contact with a greater number of professionals existed in the statutory sector than in the independent sector. (Table 4.7.)

Table 4.7
No. of different professionals keyworkers had contact with (p = >1, chi square)

	No of Establishments		
	statutory	Independent	Total
0 to 4 Different Professionals	19 (54%)	15 (65%)	34(59%)
5/5+	16 (46%)	8 (35%)	24(41%)
TOTAL (= 100%)	35	23	58

The structures to support keyworking thus appear to be located within an extensive network of contacts.

6. Matching keyworkers and service users

The literature suggests a wide range of factors that are taken into account in the process of matching. These are duplicated across many documents. For example, a typology concerning:

(i) the purpose of the placement (needs, problems, length of assistance, the care plan and possible restoration to independent living);
(ii) The previous and current experience of the client (existing relationships, age, sex, ethnic, cultural and religious factors, acceptability of the worker to the client, the previous experience of the client, and existing family ties/external influences);
(iii) the previous and current experience of the worker (age, sex, cultural and religious factors, skills, experience and training, workload and availability, relationships with other professionals and the client); and
(iv) organisational factors ((resources, workloads, time, age, sex, ethnic cultural and religious factors of all parties),

appears in RCA (1976), RCA (1978) and RCA (1983) and is quoted in Mallinson and Citarella (1990). Mallinson and Citarella extend this to also consider cultural and religious norms, and that matching as a process rather than an abstract consideration of factors. Hogan (1988) suggests the integration of role definition into RCA's approach.

The factors reported by respondents in this survey that are used in the process of matching keyworkers and service users, are now given below in the respondent's own words. In some cases the interpretation of the author is also given in brackets:

The process of matching, by:

- Mutual agreement and observation;
- Discussion and negotiation with parties concerned who then decide;
- Temperament and suitability – user choice where possible;
- Assessment and reviews of specific service user requests: and trying to accommodate
- Discussion with staff member and service user's views.
- Temporary /trial allocation;
- Staff completing a users & staff relation form/ service user choice of likes and dislikes plus ensuring a balanced workload.
- Who gets doing things with whom;
- Random selection;
- Formalisation of existing relationships;
- Availability of keyworker;
- Allocation of empty spaces;
- Trial and error;
- Geography of building (ie. presumably by aspects such as living units);
- Vacancy takes next referral;
  - Compatibility and vacancy.

Factors involved

The following aspects of factors involved were keyed directly into the process of decision-making in matching. In all cases the actual words used by the respondents are given:

- Compatablities in personalities and interests;
- More senior workers with more difficult service users;
- Gender and mixture of permanent and day care users;
- Personality, relationship – fair work load;
- Someone with knowledge of service user interests, home area, personality and approach of care assistant needs to be appropriate to service user needs;
- Needs of service user, experience/ability of keyworker + ethnic background

The actual individual factors involved are given below. Whilst the open-ended questions utilised in the questionnaire did not allow for classification, the number of establishments (out of a total number of 58 with keyworkers) where a specific factor was mentioned is given in brackets:

- Competence of staff given service user's needs (18: 38%)
- Personality and temperament (14: 24%)
  - including those of both service user and keyworker(3: 5%)
- Comparability and acceptance of both sides (13: 23%)
- Race, colour, creed,culture, language (7: 12%)
- Time given service user/ availability of staff (7: 12%)
- Attitudes and beliefs (7: 12%)
- Communication (5: 9%)
- Gender (4: 7%)
- Service user preference (4: 7%)
- Rapport (4: 7%)
- Age (3: 5%)
- Hobbies, and interests (3: 5%)
- Understanding, and empathy (2: 3%)
- Background knowledge and home situation awareness (2: 3%)
- Previous history of service user and keyworker (2: 3%)

These extend beyond the factors highlighted within the literature. There is considerable variation of approach and methodology in practice. Matching as a principle must logically be directly concerned with maintaining individualisation of the general approach to care. These results indicate that a wide variety of considered approaches to matching are extensively carried out.

7. Co-keyworking

Co-keyworking was practised in 47% of establishments in the survey with keyworker systems. There was no significant difference in the incidence of co-keyworking between sectors or size of establishment.

Mallinson and Best (1987) had suggested that co-keyworker systems increase client choice and that disadvantages of keyworker systems would be minimised by such arrangements. Whilst some factors in co-keyworking were given in this work, these represented ideas rather than researched realities of practice.

The details of co-keyworker systems given in the survey in response to an open ended question are classified and itemised below. The original wording of the respondents has been retained. Where there are more than one with the same response, the number of establishments (out of a total number of 27 with co-keyworkers) is given in brackets:

Co-keyworking based upon hierarchy

- Senior and junior staff;
- To teach juniors;
- With junior;

Co-keyworking based upon teams

- We are a small establishment, keyworkers work together;
- Based upon groups;
- Daily discussions in the staff group.
- Two teams; (3: 11%)
- Unitisation: all staff act as primary workers;

Co-keyworking based upon formal pairing

- Two senior carers work together;
- On rota basis act across for each other; (2: 7%)
- Work together in pairs, keywork for themselves and co-keywork for a colleague; (2: 7%) + discussion on a day to day basis (1)
- 2-5 keyworkers in each care group of 12 service users cover as co-keyworker when the keyworker is not on duty;
- Two keyworkers work together with four service users;
- Formally paired as backup workers;
- Two keyworkers work with six service users;
- Each unit has two co-keyworkers: cover absences

Co-keyworking based upon pragmatic arrangements

- Holiday and sick take over (4: 15%)
- Some more physically disabled service users require the help of 2 care assistants (2: 7%) + for bathing (1)

Co-keyworking is thus a particular organisational form of keyworking in which there is clearly considerable variations of practice.

8. Effect of keyworker systems

It has been suggested that keyworker systems will facilitate personalised care, relationships, and help clarify the residential task.

57 establishments (97%) in the survey with keyworkers felt that such systems improved individualised care. One (2%) felt they did not. Details are given below. The number of establishments (out of a total number of 58 with

keyworkers) where a specific enabling aspect of keyworker systems was mentioned is given in brackets.

Keyworking enabled

- Staff and service users to get to know each other as people (12: 21%)
- The fulfilment of service users' personal needs (8: 14%)
- Self esteem and dignity/ choice in dress etc. (5: 9%)
- Individualised care on a one to one basis reflecting service user choice and trust (4: 7%)
- Monitoring and reporting of any deterioration in the general wellbeing of service user (4: 7%)
- Job satisfaction and accountability (4: 7%)

48 of establishments (81%) with keyworkers felt that such systems improved relationships. One (2%) felt they did not Details are given below. The number of establishments (out of a total number of 58 with keyworkers) where a specific enabling aspect of keyworker systems was mentioned is given in brackets.

Keyworking enabled

- Getting to know each other (13: 22%)
- Enhancement of trust (9: 16%)
- Better communication (7: 12%)
- Delegation (3: 5%)
- Development of friendships with relatives

40 establishments (69%) felt that keyworker systems improved the clarity of the residential task. Six (10%) felt that they did not). Details are given below. The number of establishments (out of a total number of 58 with keyworkers) where a specific enabling aspect of keyworker systems was mentioned is given in brackets.

Keyworking enabled

- A greater knowledge of the needs of the individual (7: 12%)
- Fulfilment of aims and objectives (5: 9%)
- Decisions involving supporting, resolving and planning (5: 9%)
- Roles to be clarified (5: 9%)
- Accountability (3: 5%)
- Staff and service users to take pride in their own area (3: 5%)

36 establishments (61%) felt that keyworker systems improved other aspects of the life of the establishment. 5 (9%) felt that they did not. Details are given below. The number of establishments (out of a total number of 58 with keyworkers) where a specific enabling aspect of keyworker systems was mentioned is given in brackets.

Keyworking enabled

- A more relaxed atmosphere and job satisfaction via good relationships and networks (5: 9%)
- Attention to small but important matters, eg. buying clothes, toiletries, cigarettes, letters, going on outings (4: 7%)
- Decision-making via advocacy or counselling (3: 5%). Flexibility, recognition, responsibility and management (3: 5%)
- Identity and involvement with a member of staff to be strengthened (2: 3%)
- Healthy competition between staff to better their service (2: 3%)
- A unit to meet the needs of Asian elders quality of life

9. General comments made by respondents

Keyworking enabled

- An opportunity on both sides to build up relationships, identify needs and make goals and plans and involve relatives (2)
- The service user looks upon the keyworker as a member of their extended family
- Great changes: previously missed the finer points Staff now feel more involved in decision making
- Improved patient care (Sic)
- Achieves better job satisfaction
- Helping of officers
- Increased staff motivation by giving more responsibility and accountability and identifying training needs.

The following problem areas were also highlighted:

- Resourcing difficulties eg. a shortage of staff (sickness and annual leave) could result in a system breakdown (3)
- Needs close monitoring to check service user and staff are happy with their workload and are compatible
- Keyworkers leaving
- Part time staff may have difficulty building up relationships
- Individual service user rights lost in the system
- Constraints of level of commitment and shift system

Comments made by establishments without keyworkers:

- Not applicable in a small private home that acts as family: staff and service users are in constant communication
- The size of the home (27 service users and 30 staff <sic>) enables discussions to be made amongst us without having keyworkers – we are all keyworkers.

- Being a small home (14 service users) the senior care is the 'keyworker' she and the OIC deal with all the service users.

10. Summary and conclusions

Highlights of the findings in the survey in relation to the context of individualised care within keyworker systems in residential care for older people, are given below.

- Small group living arrangements and keyworking appear in many cases to exist side by side.
- The mean number of service users allocated to a keyworker in all establishments in the survey was 4.25.
- Race and gender were one of a number of factors involved in the matching of service users and keyworkers.
- Fewer part time staff are employed pro rata in establishments with keyworkers, thus enabling more cover to be carried out by a single full time keyworker, based upon individual relationships. The number of service users per full time equivalent staff member is higher in establishments with keyworkers.
- the tasks that keyworkers undertook in order of importance were; Physical Care, Supporting daily living, Assessment, Acting as advocate, Counselling, Admissions, Recording, Arranging activities, and Arranging outings.
- There appeared to be a wide range of networks that keyworkers link into. 91% of all keyworkers had direct contact with general practitioners, 53% with field social workers, 81% with district nurses, 74% with chiropodists and 79% with religious leaders.
- Co-keyworking was practised in 47% of establishments with keyworker systems.
- 97% of establishments with keyworkers felt that such systems improved individualised care. 81% felt they improved relationships. 69% felt they improved the clarity of the residential task. 61% felt they improved other aspects of the life of the establishment.

The exploration of the context and effect of keyworker systems, the findings of which are reported in this chapter, provided the grounding for the case explorations of keyworker practice in two individual establishments. Practice in a large statutory sector establishment is explored in the next chapter and practice in a small private sector establishment is explored in Chapter 6.

5 Painting the picture of keyworking practice: (a) The case of a large statutory establishment

This establishment was one of two, selected from the previously conducted survey, for exploration of the practice of keyworking. The keyworker system was one in which particularly interesting responses to practice requirements had been made. These are reported below using details given in interviews with keyworkers, supervisors, managers, service users and relatives. What is particularly apparent in these interview reports is the variability of practice between different keyworkers and different supervisors. Before those details are reported, the context of practice is first set by a summary of aspects of the establishment obtained from the census/survey questionnaire.

1. Setting the context: details of the establishment

The establishment had 38 service users (8 male and 30 female), all white. It also offered 6 day care places and one respite care bed. It was organised into six small living groups ranging in size from 5 service users to 17.

The following was the composition of the full time staff group (ie more than 30 hours per week) including 3 kitchen staff:

	White	Black
Male	3	1
Female	17	5

TOTAL: 26 staff plus 5 full time officer posts

In addition there were 7 part time white female staff doing over 20 but under 30 hours per week.

The establishment had a statement of aims and objectives in the form of a policy statement.

The establishment made arrangements for individual care planning through review meetings, decision-making shared between service users, relatives/friends and staff, statements or action plans, and by goal-setting formulated by staff and service users working together.

There were regular reviews (occurring at least every six months) and regular day today informal involvement of service users in decisions. In addition meetings were held where possible between care staff and the unit manager.

'Keyworkers' were said to undertake the following tasks (listed in order of importance). Generally 2/3 /a maximum of 4 service users were allocated to each keyworker.

1. Physical Care
2. Admissions
3. Assessment of residents
4. Arranging activities
5. Arranging individual outings
6. Counselling
7. Admissions
8. Recording
9. Supporting daily living

Keyworkers were supervised on a group basis. In these meetings the following methods were used: a written agreement (on approach and areas of supervision) between the supervisor and the keyworker; direction of day to day activities; a review of job responsibilities; and discussion of the service user's care plan.

Service users and keyworkers were said to be 'matched' by a simple process of direct replacement in order to maintain balance of numbers, but it was the policy of the establishment to appoint a keyworker from the first home assessment. The keyworker visited here if possible as they should have had a knowledge of the home circumstances. There was said by the officer in charge as the respondent to be the possibility of change of keyworker here as relationships may not always 'gel': 'the needs of clients vary in many ways, as care workers' abilities vary'.

Keyworkers had regular contact (ie. at least once every two months) with:

General Practitioners
Field Social Workers
District Nurses
Chiropodists

Co-keyworking was not practised.
The keyworker system was reviewed and monitored through:

Regular discussion in staff meetings;
Questionnaire /survey of service users;
Appraisal of target objectives
Supervision sessions.

In the view of the officer in charge, keyworker systems improved individualised care by 'providing the little things sometimes forgotten'; they improved relationships by 'giving a definite support and often [a] friend in strange surroundings'; they 'help with the realisation of emotional needs as well as obvious physical needs'; and they 'give a sense of added responsibility, access to outside support groups and services (day care, lunch clubs etc.) and stimulate interest'. The 'continuing involvement of relatives throughout [maintained by keyworkers] in all areas (reviews, home visits etc.) . . . ' is also important in the success of the system.

2. Themes in keyworking practice

The overall context of the keyworker system in the establishment (as described above through the census return) sets the scene for keyworker practice. Particular aspects of practice that were explored were suggested by the themes presented within the literature search. These were then formulated into a research agenda.

Explorations into the practice of individual keyworkers and their supervisors are recorded and debated below. The meaning of practice for individual service users is also considered. This is carried out by the distillation of the comments of keyworkers, supervisors, managers, service users and relatives from the interview record in relation to a number of areas of operation and considering these in relation to the debates within the literature. The themes are placed under the broad headings of relationships and decision making/meeting needs. The effect of the keyworker system is also considered:

Relationships

1. Nature of keyworker/ service user relationships
2. Relationship between keyworking and small living groups
3. How are keyworkers matched to service users?
4. Practice of co-keyworking

Decision making/meeting needs

1. Tasks undertaken by keyworkers
   - How tasks are prioritised and carried out
2. Networks: Other professionals with whom keyworkers have regular contact
3. Limitations of the role of keyworkers
4. Authority, responsibility and accountability of keyworkers,
5 How are the needs of service users met?

Effect of keyworker System

1 Effect on individualised care
2 Effect on relationships
3 Do keyworker systems clarify the residential task?

3.1 Relationships

1. Nature of keyworker/ service user relationships

In chapter two the literature search (based entirely upon theory) expressed variations between relationships founded upon sharing the companionship and friendship of mutual interests, and relationships located within a professional role. This was evident in various microcosms of practice within this establishment. Practice varied considerably between individual keyworkers. Generally speaking the focus was upon professional roles. Individual relationships involving companionship etc. existed over and above professional roles depending upon what friendships and mutual interests had been created. The main thrust of relationships between keyworkers and service users was upon offering a personalised and responsive service.

Keyworkers looked after all residents in small groups but had a particular individual responsibility for allocated service users. Three levels of professional task could be seen as operating:

general → small group → individuals as keyworkers.

Keyworkers were said to take equal care with everyone although they would pursue matters more for 'their' service users eg. clothing or outings. They provided a service based upon key tasks undertaken at quieter times in the day eg. when a service user got up, or in undertaking toileting after breakfast. A service user stated here:

You can call on any of the staff. The keyworker pops in a bit more than the other staff. If the keyworker is off sick others will ask if I want anything. In the group, its all staff and is neither here or there.

Day to day decision making appeared to be dependent upon the particular relationship between keyworker and service user. The degree of involvement here was variable. The notion of a concept of service appeared on a number of occasions when applied to day to day matters. A number of statements by keyworkers show illustrations of different individual practice philosophies affecting the nature of relationships:

Keyworkers try hard and have to respect service users. There are some strong personalities in the service user group. Keyworkers have to find out what is the truth of a matter and act regarding service user choice.

Every resident is different and communication is important . . . you know about everybody through communication . . . . A keyworker is only for bathing and special needs . . . you need to get to know all residents . . . therefore a keyworker is not special . . . . Residents wanting to be heard see their keyworker and they require action.'

It helps to know your service user and 'they' encourage areas of mutual interest . . . .

Service users tend to loose their individuality as the routine becomes the norm. Keyworkers often have too much to do to really sit down with a service user and meet other than physical needs. The rota needs to create time for this. One can do more if there is time.

One of the service users gave a particular picture of the nature of his relationship with his keyworker:

'The keyworker sees to small things and makes decisions on a day to day basis . . . . Him and me understand each other . . . little things matter as it helps the quality of life . . . . [The keyworker] helps to ask for things on my behalf.'

The relative of this service user continued this theme by stating that the keyworker and the service user worked through requirements together and the arrangement suited both of them as for example, they could decide together when bathing would take place based upon what the day's activities were for them both. In the absence of the keyworker other staff were said to also give the same service. Needs were said to be recognised by all staff but when the keyworker was there he did the looking after. Informal day to day involvement was stated by this relative to be where keyworking particularly worked well. Much of this was said to be based upon help with small things and spending time talking and chatting about events. Service user choice was said to work well here eg. whether or not they went out. The effect was 'as if he were in his own home'. There were said to be no restrictions and the keyworker enabled choice. The keyworker was said to be 'dedicated . . . nothing was too much trouble' The relative stated that in reviews this capable service user was enabled by his keyworker to put forward his needs.

Another relative commented upon 'keyworkers giving help with small things and spending time talking and chatting about events'.

A service user with learning difficulties stated 'I tend to be on my own . . . . I don't do jigsaws . . . . I see my relatives on Sundays and look forward to it . . . . I can spend time talking [to my keyworker]'. The relative of the same service user said 'the keyworker spends considerable time in a busy programme with the service user for example taking him to football matches and taking him shopping'.

The above discussion appears to relate directly to the reported experience in Burningham's establishment (1983) where 'the keyworker's task was one of helping residents to organise and enjoy their lives, to offer both care and companionship on an individual and continuous basis just as a close friend or relative might do since the act of doing something together builds up relationships.' This may now be seen as replicated, although clearly there are considerable individual practice variations.

Hopkins et al. (1984) statement that the role of the keyworker is shaped not only by the perceptions of the keyworker but by the expectations of others may also now be construed as a truism, given the interrelationship of the staff, supervisors and expectations of relatives and service users. The keyworker is part of the life space of the service user.

Tossell and Webb's (1986) description of the keyworker role as 'developing a special trusting relationship that ensures . . . a warm concern that encourages confidential communication of needs and assists . . . to develop the confidence to take an interest in a determine [the service user's] future' (p 197) may also be considered to be generally reflected in practice. It is probable that attributes of natural warmth, empathy and genuineness in a keyworker's approach to others helps to cement relationships.

Commonality of experience between residents and keyworkers as drawn out by (SCA, 1993c) is an issue that may need attention in keyworker systems, as this was again subject to considerable practice variations in this establishment. Variations between relationships founded upon sharing the companionship and friendship of mutual interests, and relationships located within a professionalised role, were extremes often present when the practice of individual keyworkers was contrasted. Generally speaking however, the focus was primarily upon professional roles. Individual relationships involving companionship etc. existed over and above professional roles depending upon what friendships and mutual interests had been created.

It may also be seen from the preceding discussion that one cannot isolate individualised care by keyworkers from the situation of group care, nor from the wider relationship with the staff team. It is useful therefore to now examine these links specifically.

2. Relationship between keyworking and small living groups

The literature search indicated that in theory, group living sets the context for keyworking given the tension that exists between individualising care and the group experience. For keyworking practice, the problem of balancing individual and collective interests was not however addressed within the literature.

The allocation of an individual keyworker implies individualised systems of care, yet users and keyworkers 'are part of a wider group within residential establishments.' (Elkan and Kelly, 1991 p 39) Thus the tension said to occur in the process of balancing individual choice against the interests of the wider residential community, is now explored. Issues indicated by the literature search to be within this theme are: how individual needs are met within the group context, the commonality of experience of residents in individualising care within a group context and the balance of individual choice and the interests of the wider residential community.

It was clear from analysis of the interviews conducted in this establishment, with managers, keyworkers, service users and relatives that (depending upon how different individual units were run) the aims of keyworking (in providing an individualised service) can however be facilitated by small group provision. Keyworking can provide a focus for small group living (eg. in terms of building relationships, enabling group interaction between service users allocated to an individual keyworker). Small group living can provide a focus for keyworking (eg. in terms of simplifying matching and allocation, enabling relationships to build up and be reciprocated, and enabling co-keyworking or similar formats for 24 hour cover and substitution during absences). The tension between individual and group needs can be worked through by individual keyworkers creating a shared view of priorities between service users and themselves. Overall however these issues appeared to need working at, as keyworking did not automatically result in these forms of practice.

According to the Officer in Charge, the keyworker system was started at about the same time as the creation of small group living areas under his predecessor some eight years prior to the time of the research interviews. Keyworking as a means of providing individualised care through named individuals linked naturally with small group living. Living areas determined allocation of keyworkers to service users as much as service user need.

To the Officer in Charge, it was clear that there was a direct link in structural terms between keyworking and small group provision (termed as 'unitisation'). Keyworkers focused within a particular work area and with a concentration of input. Small group living was said to fundamentally affect the role of keyworkers. Their responsibility and accountability was framed within small groups, needs were defined as group needs as well as individual needs.

A general input was said to be given by the keyworker and their supervisor to the group. This particularly was the case in order to ensure cover when only 2 staff would be on as a general rule at some times. The keyworker would however provide a service based upon key tasks undertaken at quieter times in the day eg. when a service user got up, or in undertaking toileting after breakfast. This structure broke down if there was sickness as the unit as a whole must then be covered.

Whilst decisions such as those concerning furniture and pictures in communal areas may have been taken in meetings concerning the whole group, individual assessment and care planning was said to be undertaken by keyworkers, in the quieter times, as a matter of course. This was based upon personal knowledge of the service user.

In the tension between individual and group needs, informal discussion between the keyworker, supervisor and service user were said to take place. Unit needs may have been decided by the supervisor (eg. day trips and equipment). Individual needs with the keyworker taking the initiative. In the day to day task these would be ad-hoc, fitting in with rotas and group needs.

The opinion of one of the supervisors was that keyworking coupled with small group living 'breaks the institutional effect (and) makes it more manageable'. The group itself was defined by needs and this helped to determine the basis of staffing. Another supervisor stated that small group living provided a family base within which to conduct keyworking. Some keyworkers were said to arrange their own co-workers but this depended upon the willingness of individual staff. A formal system had been tried on the unit but it failed because of the shift system. Care planning was said to be such that only keyworkers knew what was happening with their particular service users: others tended not to pick up 'their' care plans. There was a need to involve others but there also was a time problem here. Problems were discussed in the team but keyworkers generally tend to be isolated from the team.

Informally and on an individual basis basic tasks were said by several staff to be prioritised by keyworkers and ways of working promoted (eg. how to feed a person). The team would make decisions in every day care based upon the keyworkers input. Where there were tensions in group living (eg. where a service user wished to change dining room table, and consequently the company they would keep) the keyworker(s) was said to have a role to intervene. This was said to be based upon practical assessment and consultative ways of working. Thus individual needs were placed within a group context by the actions of those working within the keyworker system.

A relative of a service user interviewed felt that the home was too big although the groups did break it down a little (The separate lounges were said to be good and relationships in the small groups positive.) He did not know any of the staff individually. He tended to talk to whoever was on duty and was not aware of any provision through a named individual. The effect of keyworking (in terms of authority, accountability and role) was thus marginal to this particular relative.

Another of the supervisors, felt that small groups facilitated individualised service, but keyworking did not fit into this as there was friction in one unit between some keyworkers. 'Some care assistants worked well as keyworkers others were not so good.' Small group living was said to enable relationships outside the keyworker system. Friction between staff it was observed made 24 hour cover difficult as basically two groups did not get on well together. 'The rotas have to be constructed very carefully.' The supervisor maintained that in the tension between individual and group living service users allowed keyworkers time to attend to others. Sharing of activities was said to be a group phenomena as well as individual. (eg. keyworkers helping an individual make something whilst watching TV with the group.)

One of the keyworker felt that small group living is better than a big establishment. 'I have worked under both. I now take more pride in my work and know the service users better.'

A service user interviewed felt that an individualised service was given by a combination of keyworking and unitisation. In an emergency however 'they all muck in.' Allocation of keyworker just 'happened' as he was admitted in an emergency. 'You can call on any of the staff. The keyworker pops in a bit more than the other staff. If the keyworker is off sick others will ask if I want anything. In the group, its all staff and is neither here or there.' The relative of this service user commented that the particular service user tended to stay in his own room by choice and therefore small group living was not a factor. Relationships with other service users was positive. The group 'ran smoothly' as any issues had not come to a head and the keyworker had not needed to be involved. Thus the role of keyworker in individualising may have had limitations within a team approach.

The links between an individualised service and small group provision in this establishment thus appeared to be dependent upon building relationships, enabling group interaction, enabling relationships to build up and be reciprocated, and enabling formats for 24 hour cover and substitution during absences. In many cases individual keyworkers created a shared view of priorities between service users and themselves. The role as individualiser of care was in some cases limited by the team approach in others extended. What is clear from the above extracts from the interview record is the variability between individual practices. Thus accountability, responsibility and authority was often individually defined (or ill defined) depending upon the keyworker and supervisor involved. clearly this effected the nature of the relationship which was very variable.

Overall small groups living provided a focus for keyworkers meeting particular needs. and enabling communal decision making. Small groups helped communication and localising relationships, they provided a focus for keyworker decision making involving both the individual and the group.

In comparing the above practices with Bettelheim's (1974) comments upon how 'patients' and members of staff in the USA mental health group care services create their own joint commitments to fulfil special and personalised individual needs based upon deep and sensitive dyadic relationships within the context of small group living, the links between keyworking and teamwork in small group provision appear to be particularly strong where commitment and good communication is fostered. Following Mallinson (1989b), and Mallinson and Best (1987) networks of relationships would appear particularly important here in relation to decision making.

SCA's (1988/1993c) attempt to provide a formula locating keyworking firmly within the wider framework for the delivery of care via increased communication throughout residential practice including commonality of experience between residents and keyworkers appears to be particularly valid.

Links between individualised care and small group living appeared in this establishment to be dependent upon different interpretations of the task and philosophy of the establishment by the different actors in the system. The variable quality of the experience was said in the interviews to be particularly apparent. This may also be the result of variations in the quality and basis of supervision and management within the particular establishment. Different goals notionally agreed centrally appeared often to be put on one side by different supervisors. Many differences in the practice relationship of keyworking and small group living were apparent from the differing answers of the various interviewees across the five units within the establishment.

Part of linking of group and individual experience was how keyworkers were matched to service users, and how rudimentary schemes for co-working exited (in the absence of a formal scheme). These particular themes are examined next.

3. How are keyworkers matched to service users?
4. The Practice of co-keyworking

Small group living provided a focus in this establishment for matching and allocation, enabling relationships to build up and be reciprocated. Unitisation provided a focus for particular service user needs (eg. elderly mentally infirm and physical disability) and staff were matched to individual units (and therefore to specialisms eg. working with dementia). Matching to keyworkers was according to vacancies within a unit, ie. by replacement in order to maintain balance of numbers, but according to the Officer in charge, there were possibilities for change at a later date 'if they do not gel'. Small group living was said to help communication and with localising relationships. Keyworkers focused within a particular work area and with a concentration of input.

Matching of service users and keyworkers here largely follows Hogan (1988) who suggested that residents and keyworkers should be 'matched' according to the task in hand based upon an analysis of the proposed role. This is in contrast to the 'factor' based approach suggested by Mallinson and Citarella (1990), RCA/BASW (1976), and RCA (1983). Factors such as gender only occur as secondary processes in this establishment when other considerations permitted.

Small group living also provided a focus for informal co-keyworking where it occurred enabling 24 hour cover and substitution during absences. As reported in the pen picture, there was no formal co-keyworking scheme. Staff on duty took over on a random basis within small group living; the priority was to achieve cover here not to provide an individualised service. Reciprocation was practised informally, handover and administration were designed to achieve cover, although occasional friction between some staff lessened the effectiveness of systems here.

Both matching and co-working only reflect particular illustrative practices in which the context of other themes in the establishment may be assessed. Whilst it is pertinent to say that practice is based here upon linking keyworking and small group living, integrated with a team approach, no specifically firm conclusions may be attached to these explorations. For a wider exploration of the context of these themes the reader is directed back to the survey in chapter two.

3.2 Decision making/meeting needs

In this establishment, links between individual service users and formal decision – making forums are often assisted by keyworkers. Keyworkers may use decision making forums to promote individual service user's welfare by raising individual rights and general issues. In some cases, informal day to day involvement of service users in decisions may be actively pursued by keyworkers; and Keyworkers often prioritise tasks in discussion with senior staff (eg. in supervision) and by discussion with service users. The basis of decision making was found to be a fundamental part of the process of meeting needs and of the nature of the relationship between keyworkers and service users.

Levels of decision making come through clearly in the various comments of those interviewed. The three way links between keyworker, supervisor and service user were central to this. Day to day decision making appeared to be dependent upon the relationship between keyworker and service user. The degree of involvement here was variable. The notion of a concept of service appeared on a number of occasions when applied to day to day matters.

In considering the evidence for this overview, extracts from the interview record are given below.

The Officer in Charge stated that whilst all the staff on a given unit had responsibility for the service users, the keyworker had an 'extra responsibility' eg. in bathing and in purchasing small items such as toiletries. In the scope of these responsibilities there were said to be variations between units.

> In the simple day to day process of decision making the keyworker role does not have much relevance. Staff on duty have to deal with particular situations and therefore any member of staff could be involved. More complicated decisions (eg. attendance at a day centre) will involve the keyworker however. Thus the keyworker is involved where decisions may be a bit above the norm .... Where complaints may be involved, service users know that they will be acted upon. If there is a good relationship with the keyworker they will complain to them in the first instance. The keyworker will take appropriate action. Thus keyworkers are the first call in ensuring a responsive service.

As was previously explored here in relation to group living, unit needs are often decided by the supervisor (eg. day trips and equipment). In relation to individual needs the keyworker often took the initiative. In the day to day task these initiatives would be ad-hoc, fitting in with rotas and group needs. A supervisor commented here that

> ... Informally and on an individual basis ... basic tasks are prioritised by keyworkers and ways of working promoted (eg. how to feed a person). The team make decisions in every day care based upon the keyworkers input. Where there are tensions in group living (eg. where a service user wishes to change dining room table, and consequently the company they keep) the keyworker has a role to intervene. This is based upon practical assessment and consultative ways of working ....'

A keyworker involved here stated:

> Every resident is different and communication is important ... you know about everybody through communication ... [A keyworker is] only for bathing and special needs ... you need to get to know all residents ... therefore a keyworker is not special .... Residents wanting to be heard see their keyworker and they require action .... [This

> may be reflected in the] essay they want on the review. This talks about likes and dislikes. The keyworker reads it to the resident and looks at the care they are getting to get to know whether it is right.

The keyworker continued by saying that they were a filter in terms of what is important or not. 'If there is a problem we talk to the officer and they deal with it. Staff also work together'. Thus there was said by this keyworker to be a triangle of people working together in relation to tasks and decision making:

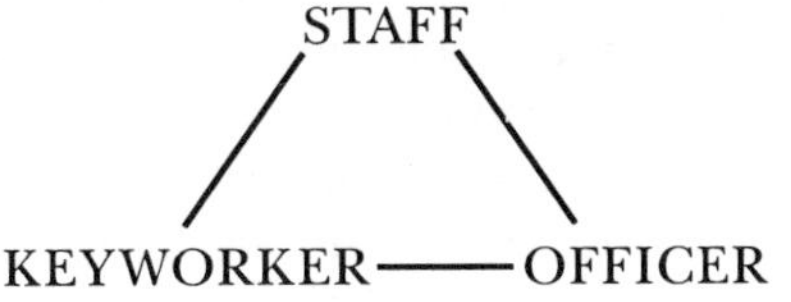

> It helps to know your service user and 'they' encourage areas of mutual interest .... Supervision every day is good, its about communication ... so as to interpret observation via discussion reaching a decision about what has to be done. Whilst its discussion together its the officer who takes the action. [In relation to relatives] some visit often then one knows them better and can answer questions but they often go to officers. They often know if there is a problem and will discuss it with the keyworker who talks to the officer. The keyworker and officer make a decision on what to do ....

Relationships appear here as in the literature to form a basis for decision making. The question of who makes the rules within relationships and within daily living in the process of keyworking in this establishment is as particularly important here as it was for Burningham (1983). The ethos in relation to roles taken by keyworkers tasks undertaken by them appears to be a particularly significant factor in the system.

As a result of analysis of the interview record, it may be said that:

- Links between individual service users and formal decision – making forums (eg. complaints procedures) may be assisted by keyworkers;

- In some cases, informal day to day involvement of service users in decisions may be actively pursued by keyworkers; and

- Keyworkers may prioritise tasks in discussion with senior staff (eg. in supervision) and by discussion with service users.

It is this focus upon the tasks of keyworkers that provides the starting point for consideration of these issues in greater depth.

1. Tasks undertaken by keyworkers, and how these tasks were prioritised and carried out

Tasks undertaken by keyworkers were considered in this study to set part of the overall context of the practice of keyworking. In this establishment, the keyworker generally took the initiative in relation to meeting individual needs. In the day to day operation these tasks would often be ad-hoc, fitting in with rotas, and team and group needs/processes. Much of the previous discussion concerning group living is directly relevant here. This part of the discussion on practice is therefore focused much more upon areas of decision making for, and meeting defined needs. The discussion that follows is therefore an illustration of how particular tasks were defined, prioritised and carried out.

The officer in charge had earlier in the census questionnaire given his view as to the tasks undertaken by keyworkers in order of priority: Physical Care; Admissions; Assessment of residents; Arranging activities; Arranging individual outings; Counselling; Admissions; Recording; and Supporting daily living. In reality, probably because it took up so much of their emotional energy, care planning and advocating needs were defined by keyworkers and supervisors as a primary part of the keyworker's role. Other responses from keyworkers indicated a focus upon bathing, purchasing toiletries, attending to practical necessities (eg. teeth, hearing aids and glasses) and involving relatives.

Whilst care planning gave a sense of focus and of structure in decision making for individual needs, it tended to be a laborious process that took a lot of each keyworker's time. Some keyworkers were very positive about the benefits it appeared to bring (in terms of involvement of users and relatives). For some keyworkers the particular process was however found stressful, eg, in writing reports. Decision making on a shared basis appeared to be enabled although the degree of choice perhaps was considerably variable (between the workers involved and the degree to which they were clear about the way the system could be used for particular purposes). The quality of the input and involvement appeared to vary according to the skills of the individual keyworker, the amount of time they freed up for individual tasks, and the degree to which they were assisted by the supervisor in understanding and achieving goals.

One supervisor commented that care planning was such that only keyworkers knew what was happening with their particular service users: others tended not to pick up their care plans. There was a need to involve others but there was a time problem here. Problems were discussed in the team but keyworkers generally tend to be isolated from the team. In the past service users were not involved in reviews and this became a hit and miss affair assessment and review was now said to firmly involve the service user. The keyworker's role was to keep the plan up to date and to set objectives via a monthly evaluation. Few if any staff focus upon this however apart from the keyworker. They would look back on an objective and see how far it had been achieved and how it should be reappraised.

The keyworker's role in care planning was thus said to involve conducting the assessment, making recommendations and then implementing the plan. (usually tangible items such as attendance at day care, tea dances or trips out). This process was said to be very dependent upon individual keyworkers.

According to the officer in charge, keyworkers investigated basic needs, made recommendations in the first instance and on discussion with the supervisor, or via a formal review, implemented a plan to meet those needs. Most inputs were said to come via the review system which would confirm need and enable moving on. Thus a crucial triangle existed here in the operation of decision making and the way tasks were defined and carried out:

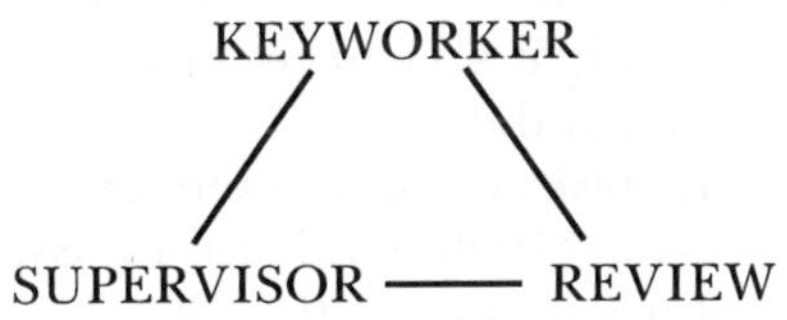

In situations where a keyworker was unavailable eg. through sickness, the function of assessment and reporting fell upon the supervisor. One keyworker said, in relation to their tasks of defining care planning needs and involving relatives:

> In care planning one needs to get to know what is happening to the resident so as to plan to meet needs . . . you look for signs and tell the officer e.g. if they are not eating or the behaviour gives rise to concern . . . . It is the officer's choice if something is done about it . . . . Residents wanting to be heard see their keyworker and they require action . . . . This may be reflected in the 'essay' they want on the review. This talks about likes and dislikes. The keyworker reads it to the resident and looks at the care they are getting to get to know whether it is right . . . . Some relative visit often then one knows them better and can answer questions but they often go to officers. They often know if there is a problem and will discuss it with the keyworker who talks to the officer. The keyworker and officer make a decision on what to do . . . . Once one knows what to do things become a matter of routine . . . we talk all the time about individual residents and any sorting out of the system comes from this . . . . Knowing ones own

residents, getting to know them and know more about their needs means that you know what they want.

The literature debates the nature of the role of keyworkers within which the tasks they undertake are founded. Ward (1978) view of the keyworker as the person responsible for 'deciding, and implementing a programme of care plus goal-directed activity specific to each resident' corresponds to practice in this establishment. RCA (1983) defined the role of keyworker in relation to individualised care planning, implementation, monitoring progress, reviews, records and maintaining relationships. The variability of individual practice that was found between different keyworkers and supervisors in this establishment partially reflects Douglas and Payne (1987) suggestion that 'each unit tends to develop its own prescription of duties for its keyworkers'. It also suggests a wider issues of training, supervision and skills development. Overall impressions indicate that the variability of keyworker practice was largely dependent upon personal capabilities of keyworkers and how much supervisors were able to manage these. Clearly the amount and quality of service given to individual service users would be dependent upon how these dimensions were handled.

The current view of the tasks of keyworkers expounded by Cambridge (1992) and Dant and Gearing (1990) ie. that they assume some direct care support for individual service users and that they have the potential to enable service user's day to day needs to be monitored and support to be provided is supported by practice in this establishment. The detailed knowledge of service users that is necessary for planning is gained through such daily contact.

The main issues in fulfilling the role and the tasks that may be involved in planning to meet needs, relate to the skills required and the support involved. It is clear that many keyworkers felt that they were not coping with the 'onerous' tasks involved in care planning, skills of report writing and assessment/ progress chasing may be maintained to be ones demanding a high degree of expertise. The variability of practice mentioned on more than one occasion probably reflected the tensions resulting from professionalisation of the care assistant's role as keyworker, and how the keyworker system was managed/ keyworkers supervised.

The process of care planning raises the question of contact with other professionals. That is the next theme to be explored.

2. Networks: other professionals with whom keyworkers have regular contact

Whilst keyworkers in this establishment had regular contact (ie. at least once every two months) with: General Practitioners, Field Social Workers, District Nurses, and Chiropodists, the focus here tended to be on the basis of reporting for reviews and routine/ emergency medical treatment. In many instances this contact was carried out in practice by supervisors on a routine basis. Virtually all persons interviewed saw contact with relatives as the main networking role of keyworkers.

Relatives were seen by the officer in charge to be a mouthpiece for the service user to develop the theme of what the service user wanted.

> Clients still feel threatened [by the formal nature of the review proceedings and they] do not necessarily know what a review is . . . Relatives are invited to reviews and the keyworkers involvement with them is crucial. It is vital to create the right input . . . relatives may control the cash flow for extra resources for a particular resident . . . . An example of keyworker involvement in the family network was when a keyworker handled a resident's input (present, dress and attendance) at her daughter's wedding . . . . Negotiation with relatives of the resident's care plan may be a rewarding or frustrating role for keyworkers. It is the framework for relationships . . . . Keyworkers give the report to the review and this is an indication to the relative of what has to be done.

Many of the natural relatives were said to have withdrawn from regular contact although keyworkers enjoyed good relationships with relatives who could be encouraged by them to attend reviews and give support. One keyworker stated:

> Some visit often then one knows them better and can answer questions but they often go to officers. They often know if there is a problem and will discuss it with the keyworker who talks to the officer. The keyworker and officer make a decision on what to do . . . . Once one knows what to do things become a matter of routine . . . we talk all the time about individual residents and any sorting out of the system comes from this . . . . Knowing one's own residents, getting to know them and know more about their needs means that you know what they want.

The relative referred to stated however that he tended to talk to whoever was on duty and was not aware of any provision through a named individual. Contact with staff was thus general and tended to stay around general issues.

A supervisor commented:

> . . . Some links with relatives by keyworkers are very good, discussions take place about all aspects of care. This may however be a function of the length of time that a keyworker has been in role and how frequent a relative will visit. In the implementation of the care plan relatives

may be asked for help and encouragement. This is achieved with variable success. The keyworker may take action to make things happen eg. to sit with relatives It is a question of both taking time to know the finer details of likes and dislikes and to really get to know the service user.

A Keyworker from the same unit stated that they get to know relatives.

> It is very important to deal with things if they are upset and to see how they are feeling so that they can do things for the service user. The family is involved in care planning as the relationship can affect the service user. Keyworkers promote the quality of the relationship but care planning is not really discussed with them except in relation to reviews . . . . The family often approach staff. The supervisor and keyworker acting together see the family. This works well there are close bonds. If there is no family at all loneliness can be the result. The keyworker's job is to be closer and to compensate for this . . . . Care planning is discussed at every staff meeting but it is too complicated and too much writing other areas are not then discussed. The system based on care planning is not relevant [to meeting needs].

A relative commented here that the keyworker's links with relatives worked well. As a result they did much to contribute to the establishment. The keyworker would often contact them and although the service user was very independent when things gave rise for concern the relatives and keyworker would talk them through.

Another keyworker said,

> . . . Contact with relatives takes place mainly when they visit. They let you know how a service user is getting on. and what they want to do . . . . The effect of keyworking is more contact and relationships based upon trying to deal with problems. Those you look after you get to know more. (It) helps care planning and if something needs to be done . . . one makes sure every one else knows. Communication is important . . . one knows their needs more . . . things are clearer.

A relative of a service user also commented that the review was a key point of action between the relative, service user and the keyworker as representative of the establishment. In deciding what had to be done contact between relative and keyworker/ supervisor was fundamental. Home visits were arranged via this contact.

Suggestions by Cambridge (1992) and Dant and Gearing (1990) that keyworkers in residential care now (in addition to their direct caring role) need to liaise closely with decision makers, feeding information directly into IPP or case reviews, or indirectly via other workers such as case/care managers. Appear embryonic in the practice of this establishment.

The area of contact with and involvement of relatives is however totally neglected in the literature on keyworking. Following the discussion within this section the issues that apply within this case study may be summarised as:

- principles involved in the discussion and talking through of the care plan with relatives;
- participation roles in family events;
- role of supervisor appropriate in relation to keyworking activities; jointness, and respective boundaries;
- principles involved in the involvement of relatives in the day to day tasks of care;
- Appropriateness of role of keyworker as a 'substitute family member'.

All these issues have a common focus upon the role of keyworkers which is the theme to be explored next.

3. Limitations of the role of keyworkers

The boundaries of the keyworker's role in this establishment are formulated with and defined by their relationship with service users, the staff team, and with their supervisor. This thread may be seen running through the preceding discussion of the other themes. For example, the team would make decisions in every day care based upon the keyworkers input.

These kind of boundaries between the team and between supervisors/keyworkers may vary between workers depending upon their skills. One of the supervisors, felt here that 'Some care assistants worked well as keyworkers others were not so good.' The primary responsibility of the keyworker was said to be care planning, a process they were accountable within. The system was a primary part of defining needs of service users to be met. The fundamental issue for the keyworker system was however the variability in approach and the degree to which supervisors were responsible rather than keyworkers. The role of keyworkers was in theory well defined in practice it was diffuse and variable. This clearly must affect questions of accountability of keyworkers and the relationships between keyworkers and service users.

The boundary between keyworkers and supervisors had to be discussed in order to define it and make it work. Keyworkers in prioritising tasks did so in discussion with senior staff (e.g. in supervision) and by discussion with service users. The practice here was extremely variable. One supervisor commented for example: 'The role of the supervisor is to try to guide the keyworker.' One keyworker stated: 'Important decisions are taken by officers, supervision is given in occasional unit meetings.'

Similarly the boundaries in the care process between relatives, service user and keyworkers were individually formulated. A relative stated that the keyworker and the service user worked through requirements together and the arrangement suited both of them as for example, they could decide together when bathing would take place based upon what the day's activities were for them both. In the absence of the keyworker other staff were said to also give the same service.

A flexibly defined role will only work (it may be maintained) if conflict is avoided by working through issues. This appears to have been the case in this establishment. These is still the question of the variable effect of practice between different keyworkers and the potential for some areas to be neglected unless systems are in place and there is clear agreement in supervision of respective roles and responsibilities.

The debate of this question makes clear that role cannot be isolated from that of authority, responsibility, and accountability. These are to be explored next.

4. Authority, responsibility and accountability of keyworkers

Analysis of the previously reported and discussed interview record indicates that the role of keyworkers in this establishment was in theory well defined yet in practice it was diffuse and variable. This clearly must affect questions of accountability of keyworkers and the relationships between keyworkers and service users. Keyworkers were generally said to be accountable through supervision to the head of the unit they worked within. Informal accountability was to relatives.

Where a keyworker states however that they are a filter in terms of what is important or not, the clear question is how they determine what is important. The keyworker continued: 'If there is a problem I talk to the officer and they deal with it. Staff also work together'. There appeared to be no clear criteria as to where these boundaries lay only custom and practice. Such custom and practice varied between different keyworkers and different supervisors.

In the establishment the team would make decisions in every day care based upon the keyworkers input. This was affected by variations in the quality and basis of supervision and management within the establishment. The role as individualiser of care was in some cases limited by the team approach in others extended. There were variability between individual practices. Problems were discussed in the team but keyworkers generally tend to be isolated from the team.

In addition there were different interpretations of the task and philosophy of the establishment by the different actors in the system. Different goals notionally agreed centrally appeared often to be put on one side by different supervisors. Accountability, responsibility and authority were often individually defined (or ill defined) depending upon the keyworker and supervisor involved.

The team made decisions in every day care based upon the keyworkers input. They were a filter in terms of what is important or not. Needs were said to be recognised by all staff but when the keyworker was there they did the looking after.

These issues mirror discussion by Davis (1978) who expressed the organisational problems and constraints that had become significant given ambiguities in the keyworker 'concept'. He specifically mentions 'the shadow of accountability . . . [and] . . . divided loyalties' in the context of confidentiality, communication, and power in/ the power of relationships. The variability of practice was also clear to Davis who in contrast quoted situations where keyworkers had developed relationships with service users of such quality that they became totally available and involved as advocates for service user's rights and champions in individualised development. Davis (1978) and this study highlights here a basic issue, that as a decision maker, a keyworker can only be as good as other workers and the system would allow.

SCA (1992b) states that keyworking in residential care for older people provides a structure. Responsibility, accountability and decision-making appear to be issues here that require additional formulation if a system is to work well. The implementation of sound principles of individualised care is clearly dependent upon this.

5. How are the needs of service users met?

As we have already seen in the preceding discussion, different interpretations of the task and philosophy of the establishment by the different actors in the system result in variable keyworker-service user relationships and quality and effect of decision making. This is partially the result of variations in the quality and basis of supervision and management within the establishment. Different goals notionally agreed centrally appeared often to be put on one side by different supervisors and then by different keyworkers.

Part of these variations occur between units (inevitably perhaps, as units have different supervisors). Unitisation also provided a focus for particular service user needs (eg. elderly mentally infirm and physical disability) and as we have seen staff were matched to individual units according to specialisms such as working with dementia. Needs were defined as group needs as well as individual needs. Unit needs were often decided by the supervisor (eg. day trips and equipment). Keyworkers taking the initiative with individual needs on an ad-hoc basis, fitting in with rotas and between meeting group needs.

As we have seen the main way of defining needs to be met was through care planning. This was seen as a primary part of the keyworker role. Some keyworkers were very positive about the benefits care planning brought in terms of involvement of users and relatives. Decision making on a shared basis appeared to be enabled although the degree of choice perhaps was considerably variable (between the workers involved and the degree to which they were clear about the way the system could be used for particular purposes). The quality of the input and involvement appeared to vary according to the skills of the individual keyworker and the degree to which they were assisted by the supervisor in understanding and achieving those goals. Where links with relatives were particularly meaningful the system provided a clear focus for meeting needs and implementing plans devised for that purpose.

The Officer in Charge stated that regular discussions would take place between keyworker, supervisor and service user. A review would then take place after two weeks and thereafter at three monthly intervals. The keyworker's role involved conducting the assessment, making recommendations and then implementing the plan. (usually tangible items such as attendance at day care, tea dances or trips out). There was said to be no pressure on service users and their views were listened to carefully by the individual keyworker who has a responsibility to spend time 'chatting' to service users in order to assess their lifestyle needs and the import of possible decision making options.

Keyworkers investigated basic needs, made recommendations in the first instance and on discussion with the supervisor, or via a formal review, implemented a plan to meet those needs. In situations where a keyworker was unavailable eg. through sickness, the function of assessment and reporting fell upon the supervisor.

One of the supervisors commented that the process of care planning was one in which the keyworker and supervisor would jointly talk and assess based upon observations (eg. of the service user's need for security) although it was the keyworker's task in the review process to initiate and take action. Relatives needs were also said to be part of an assessment. Facilities were offered based upon interpretation of wishes. Keyworkers, it was said, needed to observe in order to respond and interpret. Needs were thought about by keyworkers and constructively put on paper. This it was maintained enabled them to get beyond thinking about physical care. The central issues was the service user as a person. The time involved with this process was said to be a problem given other demands upon it. A keyworker stated that:

> In care planning one needs to get to know what is happening to the resident so as to plan to meet needs . . . you look for signs and tell the officer e.g. if they are not eating or the behaviour gives rise to concern . . . . It is the officer's choice if something is done about it . . . . Residents wanting to be heard see their keyworker and they require action . . . . This may be reflected in the 'essay' they want on the review. This talks about likes and dislikes. The keyworker reads it

to the resident and looks at the care they are getting to get to know whether it is right.

The same keyworker continued by talking about relatives:

> Some visit often then one knows them better and can answer questions but they often go to officers. They often know if there is a problem and will discuss it with the keyworker who talks to the officer. The keyworker and officer make a decision on what to do . . . . Once one knows what to do things become a matter of routine . . . we talk all the time about individual residents and any sorting out of the system comes from this . . . . Knowing ones own residents, getting to know them and know more about their needs means that you know what they want.

Another supervisor commented,

> 'Keyworkers try hard and have to respect service users . . . . service users will say what they want. It is the keyworkers task to write the paperwork to enable this . . . . Some links with relatives by keyworkers are very good discussions take place about all aspects of care. This may however be a function of the length of time that a keyworker has been in role and how frequent a relative will visit. In the implementation of the care plan relatives may be asked for help and encouragement. This is achieved with variable success. The keyworker may take action to make things happen e.g. to sit with relatives. It is a question of both taking time to know the finer details of likes and dislikes and to really get to know the service user.

A Keyworker from the same unit stated that,

> We get to know the relatives. It is very important to deal with things if they are upset and to see how they are feeling so that they can do things for the service user. The family is involved in care planning as the relationship can affect the service user. Keyworkers promote the quality of the relationship but care planning is not really discussed with them except in relation to reviews . . . . The family often approach staff. The supervisor and keyworker acting together see the family. This works well there are close bonds. If there is no family at all loneliness can be the result. The keyworker's job is to be closer and to compensate for this . . . . Care planning is discussed at every staff meeting but it is 'too complicated and too much writing' other areas are not then discussed. The system based on care planning is not relevant [to meeting needs].

In another unit, the supervisor commented that care planning was such that,

> Only keyworkers know what was happening with their particular service users: others tended not to pick up their care plans. There was a need to involve others but there was a time problem here. Problems were discussed in the team but keyworkers generally tend to be isolated from the team. In the past service users were not involved in reviews and this became a hit and miss affair assessment and review was now said to firmly involve the service user. The keyworker's role was to keep the plan up to date and to set objectives via a monthly evaluation. Few if any staff focus upon this however apart from the keyworker. They would look back on an objective and see how far it had been achieved and how it should be reappraised.

A keyworker involved here amplified this by saying that,

> Care planning tended to be 'elaborate' keyworkers concentrated on the situation and make recommendations as to how they are dealt with so as to improve things. The keyworkers fill in the forms monthly. This helps to sort out priorities . . . . Contact with relatives takes place mainly when they visit. They let you know how a service user is getting on. and what they want to do . . . . The effect of keyworking is more contact and relationships based upon trying to deal with problems. Those you look after you get to know more. It helps care planning and if something needs to be done . . . one makes sure every one else knows. Communication is important . . . one knows their needs more . . . things are clearer'.

Thus a sense of focus for meeting needs by keyworkers appeared to be generated by care planning. Care planning activities appeared to give assistance in enabling promotion of shared decision – making and service user choice. Some keyworkers actively created links between persons involved in the care process (eg. relatives) in order to implement the service user's care plan. Evaluative questions regarding the effectiveness of these processed of defining and meeting needs were not however addressed in the interviews. Although it appears that all concerned (including service users and relatives) found care planning helpful and the outcomes beneficial, the question of whether this particular care planning system was the most efficient in meeting needs and whether there might be alternative formulations of practice was not the brief of this study.

The importance of internal/external care planning to define needs and ways of meeting them in residential care has been recognised for some time. Ward (1978) discussed the the keyworker as the person responsible for 'deciding, and implementing a programme of care plus goal-directed activity specific to each resident'. These are the main features of planning and progressing/ coordinating care as promoted within this system. The central role of the keyworker as utilised here is reflected throughout the literature promoting keyworker systems. For example, RCA (1983) defined the role in meeting individualised needs as care planning, implementation, monitoring progress, reviews, records and maintaining relationships.

Nonetheless, in this establishment, different interpretations of the semantics of the care planning task and its philosophy by different keyworkers and supervisors must result in variable keyworker-service user relationships and quality and effect of decision making. The operation of the care planning system is dependent upon differential interpretations of the role and practice of keyworkers. The generation of effective skills that are involved may not have a consistency across all the keyworkers and the quality of the particular relationship will affect the ability of some service users to fully participate. The quality of care planning is also dependent upon other factors such as, for example, how much relatives participate or do not participate in the process, this again raises questions regarding the effectiveness of individual keyworkers and their interpretation of their role.

If care planning and involvement of relatives in the context of relationships between service users and keyworkers is construed as the main basis of keyworker practice in this establishment, the question of the effect of these and of the keyworker system as a whole may now be raised.

4. Summary: effect of this keyworker system

By way of a summary a number of factors may be stated in relation to the effect of this keyworker system:

1. Individualised care

- Group needs as well as individual needs were framed within the system.

- Individual needs were placed within a group context by the actions of those working within the keyworker system.

- An individualised service was given by a combination of keyworking and unitisation.

- The quality of the input and involvement appeared to vary according to the skills of the individual keyworker and the degree to which they were assisted by the supervisor in understanding and achieving those goals.

- Input to reviews was conducted entirely through keyworkers. Needs were assessed by keyworkers. This it was maintained enabled them to get beyond thinking about physical care.

- Keyworker and the service users often worked through requirements together deciding what the day's activities were for them both.

- Needs were recognised by all staff but when the keyworker was there they initiated the main care inputs.

- Keyworkers enabled service user to put forward their needs and requirements.

- Different levels of individualised decision making occur in keyworker practice. Discussions between keyworker, supervisor and service user are notable in framing this.

- Keyworkers would pursue matters more for 'their' service users – The keyworker's role in care planning was to conduct the assessment, make recommendations and then implement the agreed plan.

- The team made decisions in every day care based upon the keyworkers input. They were a filter in terms of what is important or not. Needs were said to be recognised by all staff but when the keyworker was there they did the looking after.

2. Relationships

- Keyworking can build relationships, enabling group interaction – Responsibility and accountability for individualising care was framed within within small groups.

- Keyworking coupled with small group living was said to 'break the institutional effect'.

- Small groups were defined by common needs. This determined the basis of staffing and keyworker relationships.

- Small group living provided a family base within which keyworking was conducted. Small group living helped communication enabling relationships to build up and be reciprocated.

- Problems were discussed in the team but keyworkers generally tend to be isolated from the team.
- Small group living enabled relationships outside the keyworker system.
- Sharing of activities was a group phenomena as well as individual. (eg. keyworkers helping an individual make something whilst watching TV with the group.)
- A fundamental issue was the variability in approach and the degree to which supervisors were responsible rather than keyworkers. The variability in the role of keyworkers was thought to affect the relationships between keyworkers and service users.
- Keyworking can build relationships, enabling group interaction.
- Links were made with relatives by keyworkers in order to implement the individual service user's care plan.
- Day-to-day decision making appears dependent upon the quality of the individual relationship between keyworker and service user.
- Sharing of areas of mutual interest between keyworker and service users appeared to be framed by the individual relationship and support given by supervisors.
- Accountability, responsibility and authority were often individually defined (or ill defined) depending upon the keyworker and supervisor involved.

3. Clarity of the residential task

- Keyworkers provide a service based upon a task focus within small group living.
- The quality of the input and involvement appeared to vary according to the skills of the individual keyworker and the degree to which they were assisted by the supervisor in understanding and achieving those goals.
- Keyworkers and supervisors would often jointly consider situations, although it was the keyworker's task in the review process to initiate and take action.

- A fundamental issue was the variability in approach and the degree to which supervisors were responsible rather than keyworkers.

- The role of keyworkers was in theory well defined, in practice it was diffuse and variable.

- The creation of shared view of priorities between service users and keyworkers occurred. Practice here varied according to the particular keyworker.

- Care planning through keyworkers gave focus and a sense of structure to providing for individual needs. The quality of the input and involvement appeared here to vary according to the skills of the individual keyworker and the degree to which they were assisted by the supervisor.

- Links were made with relatives by keyworkers in order to implement the individual service user's care plan.

- Day to day decision making appears dependent upon the quality of the individual relationship between keyworker and service user.

- Sharing of areas of mutual interest between keyworker and service users appeared to be framed by the individual relationship and support given by supervisors.

- Meeting the needs of service users through keyworking was affected by different interpretations of the task and philosophy of the establishment.

- Keyworkers would pursue matters more for 'their' service users – Small group living provided a focus for general needs.

- Care Planning as a primary part of the keyworker role gave a focus and a sense of structure to providing for individual needs. – The keyworker's role in care planning was to conduct the assessment, make recommendations and then implement the agreed plan.

- The team would make decisions in every day care based upon the keyworkers input.

- There were three levels of decision making operating in the establishment: general → small group → individuals as keyworkers. This was affected by variations in the quality and basis of supervision and management within the establishment.

- The role of keyworkers as individualiser of care was in some cases limited by the team approach in others extended. There were variability between individual practices. Problems were discussed in the team but keyworkers generally tend to be isolated from the team.

- The role of keyworkers was in theory well defined, but in practice it was diffuse and variable.

- There were different interpretations of the task and philosophy of the establishment by the different actors in the system. Different goals notionally agreed centrally appeared often to be put on one side by different supervisors.

5. Conclusions

The particular *strengths* of this keyworker system in contributing towards improved individualised care may be said to involve:

- Individual needs being framed within the group context and the small living unit.

- The keyworker role focusing upon care planning, giving a structure linking relationships and meeting needs.

- Keyworker and the service users work together on requirements and decisions.

- Every day care was a team function based upon the keyworkers input.

- Building relationships and enabling group interaction.

- Responsibility and accountability was generally clear.

- Purposeful relationships could be build up and be reciprocated.

- Links made with relatives by keyworkers in order to implement the individual service user's care plan.

- The creation of shared view of priorities between service users and keyworkers occurred.

The *weaknesses* of this particular keyworker system in terms of its ability to contribute towards improved individualised care may be said to involve:

- The quality of the input and involvement of the keyworker varying according to the individual involved.
- Supervision being variable in quality and effect.
- Although problems were discussed in the team, keyworkers generally tended to be isolated from the team.
- The variability in the role of keyworkers effected some relationships between keyworkers and service users.
- Sharing between keyworker and service users appeared to be framed by the individual relationship and by support given by supervisors.
- Accountability, responsibility and authority were often variably defined depending upon the keyworker and supervisor involved.
- The role of keyworkers was in theory well defined, in practice it was often diffuse and variable.
- The quality of the input and involvement of the keyworker in care planning appeared here to vary according to the skills of the individual keyworker and the degree to which they were assisted by the supervisor.
- Day to day decision making appears dependent upon the quality of the individual relationship between keyworker and service user.
- Meeting the needs of service users through keyworking was affected by different interpretations of the task and philosophy of the establishment.
- Different goals notionally agreed centrally appeared often to be put on one side by different supervisors.

The question may be asked whether these are strengths and weaknesses of keyworker systems in general, or only of this particular keyworker system. In an endeavour to begin to answer this question, keyworking in a different establishment will be examined so that subsequent comparisons may be made. The next chapter considers a further case study in a different establishment.

6 Painting the picture of keyworking practice: (b) The case of a small private sector establishment

This establishment was the second of two selected as previously detailed from the survey, for exploration of the practice of keyworking. Reported below are details given in interviews with keyworkers, supervisors, managers, service users and relatives. What is again apparent in these interview reports is the variability of practice between different keyworkers and different supervisors.

The terminology employed in the establishment for keyworker was 'primary carer'. The terms 'primary carer' and 'keyworker' have therefore been used interchangeably. (Where a persons actual title is referred to, or verbatim quotes made, 'primary carer' has been used; where interpretive statements are made, the term 'keyworker' is employed.)

Before details of practice are reported, its context is first set by a summary of aspects of the establishment obtained from the census/survey questionnaire.

1. Setting the context: details of the establishment

The establishment had 25 service users (4 male, 21 female) all white. It had 3 day care places and offered respite care as available. It was organised into 3 living groups each of approximately 8 service users.

The composition of the full time staff group (i.e. more than 30 hours per week) including domestic staff was as follows:

	White	Black
Male	2	–
Female	15	6

TOTAL: 26 staff plus 5 full time officer posts

In addition there were 6 part time staff (4 white female and 2 black females) doing less than 10 hours per week and four white females doing 10-20 hours per week.

The establishment was said to have statements of aims and objectives in the forms of a prospectus, a policy statement, a charter of rights and a document for discussion.

The establishment made arrangements for individual care-planning through review meetings, contracts /agreements, decision-making shared between service users, relatives/friends and staff, and by goal setting formulated by staff and service users working together.

There was a regular users' committee (meeting at least once per month), regular staff/ service users meetings (meeting at least once per month), regular reviews (occurring at least every six months) and regular day to day informal involvement of service users in decisions.

'Prime Carers' undertook the following tasks (listed in order of importance) with one service user only allocated to each.

1. 'Sitting and listening to residents joys and worries etc.'
2. Admissions
3. Assessment of residents
4. Advocating resident's needs
5. Physical care
6. Counselling
7. Recording
8. Supporting daily living
9. Arranging individual outings
10. Arranging activities

All staff including the housekeeper, the laundry assistant and the management team were involved in the role of keyworking/prime caring.

Keyworkers were supervised on a daily basis by the following methods: direction of day to day activities; review of job responsibilities and discussion of the service user's care plan.

Service users and keyworkers were matched by the following factors: 'personality, disability, age and sex.'

Keyworkers had regular contact (i.e. at least once every two months) with:

General Practitioners
District Nurses
Chiropodists
Religious leaders
'Solicitors and family of residents.'

Co-keyworking was practised on a 'rota basis act[ing] across for each other.'

The keyworker system was reviewed and monitored through supervision sessions.

In the view of the Director of Care, keyworker systems improved individualised care by giving an 'interest to the keyworker'. Relationships were 'like an extended family' whilst 'staff are aware of their responsibility and their aims and objectives . . . . The keyworker is able to keep family and relatives up to date, write letters etc. if necessary arrange birthday parties, (and) send cards to relatives on (the) resident's behalf'.

2. Themes in keyworking practice

The overall context of the keyworker system in the establishment (as described above through the census return) sets the scene for keyworker practice. Particular aspects of practice that were explored were suggested by the themes presented within the literature search. These were then formulated into a research agenda.

Explorations into the practice of individual keyworkers and their supervisors are recorded and debated below. The meaning of practice for individual service users is also considered. This is carried out by the distillation of the comments of keyworkers, supervisors, managers, service users and relatives from the interview record in relation to a number of areas of operation and considering these in relation to the debates within the literature. The themes are placed under the broad headings of relationships and decision making/meeting needs. The effect of the keyworker system is also considered:

Relationships

1. Nature of keyworker/ service user relationships

2. Relationship between keyworking and small living groups

3. How are keyworkers matched to service users?

4. Practice of co-keyworking

Decision making/meeting needs

1. Tasks undertaken by keyworkers
   - How tasks are prioritised and carried out

2. Networks: Other professionals with whom keyworkers have regular contact

3. Limitations of the role of keyworkers

4. Authority, responsibility and accountability of keyworkers,

5. How are the needs of service users met?

Effect of keyworker system

1. Effect on individualised care

2. Effect on relationships

3. Do keyworker systems clarify the residential task?

3.1 Relationships

1. Nature of keyworker/ service user relationships

A focus for small group living was provided by keyworking in this establishment, in terms of building relationships, and in enabling group interaction between service users allocated to individual keyworkers. Small group living provided a focus for keyworker allocation, and in enabling relationships to build up and be reciprocated. Relationships were generally said to involve trust, providing services and making service users content and feeling at home.

According to the Director of Care, keyworking or 'primary care' was based upon developing relationships and trust. A service user's relative said that working with a small number of persons enabled staff to exhibit empathy and tolerance. The quality of the relationship between a keyworker and an individual service user was said to be of considerable importance when needs may not be readily apparent due to the service user's confusion.

A supervisor who was also primary carer commented:

> Primary carers can see if service users are having a problem and can talk about it in confidence. They do not take over but go with them .... Expectations are based upon mutual trust .... Relationships frame the analysis of needs. The prime carer will need to know all their service users very well and if something is not right pick it up ... [examples here were said to be if they were unwell or feelings of unease when their family were away on holiday] .... If a service user is not

> happy with an issue they will say so . . . . In sorting out priorities the prime carer will talk to their supervisor. Flexibility is the keynote. They will try to do what the service user wants . . . .

This professional view of the relationship was not shared by all staff. Indeed many keyworkers presented a different view of the way relationships evolved within a task focus. The tension appeared to exist whether relationships concerned companionship/friendship or such focused intervention. For example, one primary carer stated:

> They have a joke, a chat and a moan . . . it differs every night . . . I share interests with them e.g. sharing family events and stories from the past.

Another primary carer said:

> Day to day its via relationships enabling communication. There is a continual focus on service users on their comfort and well being. We go and see them and if they are OK when we are in.

In some instances keyworkers would seek to promote areas of mutual interests between themselves and service users (e.g. hobbies). The Director of Care stated that the prime carer would 'share in the service user's life space, as they read talk and listen'. The prime carer, it was said, would see their family and organise social outings. The relationship factor the Director maintained was vitally important.

Inputs appeared to vary according to the particular keyworker and the relationship they may have with the service user (and relatives). Thus the amount that they are 'part of the service user's life space' varied. The question as to who defined the nature of this life space is unanswered in the data. It may also be asked how much outings and stimulation were part of the formal mechanisms of care (i.e. planned for as part of a 'treatment' programme) and how much was informal like a 'chat and a moan'.

The main dimensions concerning relationships that are present in the literature on keyworking appear within this establishment. Burningham (1983) for example saw the keyworker's task as one of helping residents to organise and enjoy their lives, to offer both care and companionship on an individual and continuous basis just as a close friend or relative might do. This tallies with much of the espoused practice of keyworking in here. Indeed the idea of 'the special relationship' between the worker and service user (Rodway, 1981) may now be considered in relation to overall group interaction. The view of Hopkins et al. (1984) who state that the role of the keyworker is shaped not only by the perceptions of the keyworker but by the expectations of others, with the keyworker seen as part of the life space of the service user is a common thread in practice here (although variable in the extent to which it applies). It may be confirmed in practice that Keyworkers are said to need the attributes of natural warmth, empathy and genuineness in their approach to others.

The view expressed in SCA (1993c) that commonality of experience between residents and keyworkers may be an issue in the variability of practice, appears to be borne out in the data.

The ambiguity contained elsewhere in the literature concerning relationships, i.e. whether they are based upon sharing the companionship and friendship of mutual interests, or based entirely upon a professionalised role appears to evolve entirely here into the practice of individual keyworkers and their supervisors. There is not one interpretation that fully holds for the practice throughout this establishment. This must be considered to create a differential effect in practice for different service users and their relationships with staff.

Overall relationships of quality appear to be promoted here. The question mark concerns variability in their foundation and purpose particularly relative to possible differential interpretations of task.

2. Relationship between keyworking and small living groups

There appeared to be a direct link between keyworking and small group living in this establishment. The living areas were fluid rather than rigid entities. The aims of keyworking (in providing an individualised service) appeared to be facilitated by small group provision. A focus for small group living was provided by keyworking (in terms of building relationships, and in enabling group interaction between service users allocated to an individual keyworker).

Small group living in many cases provided a focus for keyworking, in allocation, and in enabling relationships to build up and be reciprocated. The tension between individual and group needs could be worked through by individual keyworkers creating a shared view of priorities between service users and themselves.

According to the Director of Care, a creative view of the task was taken but was independent of small groups. The establishment focused on small group living through interlinked lounges. The 'sitting rooms' were graded according to dependency. Living areas were not rigid but, the Director said, developed by custom and practice. There was an interlinking between areas of the establishment. The group was said tend to dominate in day to day living, tensions were worked through by discussion however. It was suggested that there was always the possibility of personal space in the service user's own room.

A particular primary carer commented as a member of the night shift:

> I have a wider responsibility for three small groups but have primary carer responsibility for five of the twenty five service users. I was allocated these five because they had particular needs on the night shift . . . .

Another primary carer who was a housekeeper /laundry assistant stated that small group provision allowed day to day needs to be met. Differences in needs were, she said, particularly apparent in the primary care role, as 'one goes into them deeper . . . one needs to get to know them.' She appeared particularly aware of relationship needs.

A service user's relative said that small group living created a sense of focus and enabled the staff to work with a small number of persons.

A primary carer who was a senior care on the night shift stated that their work was across all groups but as primary carer, they tended to concentrate on the one lounge where the particular service users are allocated. Thus it was said that small group living provided a particular focus for activities on the shift. In the tension between group and individual living the primary carer she suggested, could also be the adjudicator in any arguments, although she stated that on nights this did not tend to come into the fore.

It may be said that in this establishment:

- the aims of keyworking (in providing an individualised service) may be facilitated by small group provision;
- keyworking can provide a focus for small group living (e.g. in terms of building relationships, enabling group interaction between service users allocated to an individual keyworker);
- small group living can provide a focus for keyworking (e.g. in terms of simplifying matching and allocation, enabling relationships to build up and be reciprocated, and enabling co-keyworking or similar formats for 24 hour cover and substitution during absences); and that
- the tension between individual and group needs may be worked through by individual keyworkers creating a shared view of priorities between service users and themselves.

Practice did however vary considerably between different keyworkers and their supervisors.

Practice elaborated in Bettelheim (1974) tallies with that discussed above, in that members of staff create their own joint commitments to fulfil special and personalised individual needs based upon deep and sensitive dyadic relationships within the context of small group living. Following Bromley (1977) the quality of interaction appears also to be a significant factor in relation to forming individual and group relationships.

The issue of balancing individual and collective interests appears to evolve into the particular practices of individual keyworkers and supervisors. In the tension between individualised systems of care and needs of the wider group, the overall impression gained in this establishment is that in most cases individual choice is the province of keyworkers and supervisors, whilst interests of the wider residential community appears to be defined by the senior management of the establishment, as personified by the Director of Care. Part of the variation in practice therefore results from the fact that practitioners, first line managers and senior managers all take on (to a greater or lesser extent) a keyworking role. Non the less, the interviews point to positive relationships here within the keyworker system, in the context of the small group experience.

3. How are keyworkers matched to service users?
4. The practice of co-keyworking

The Director of Care stated that, matching of prime carers was creatively based upon developing relationships i.e. 'whoever gets on with whom. The service user states who they wish their prime carer to be. They have the choice of the person they get on well with. If a service user is confused, the staff will chose for them based upon the relationships in progress'.

A supervisor who was also primary carer commented that the head of care decided on matching. The supervisor said that the head tried to do this according to personalities and the ability of the carer to appreciate a particular service user's problems.

This approach to matching generally reflects that based on 'factors'. Those factors particularly involved were personality, disability, age and sex. In the literature this method accords with RCA (1983) and Mallinson and Citarella (1990) In particular the process involved is discussed in Mallinson and Citarella in the way that feelings and emotions of service users are important issues as utilised herein.

In relation to co-working, the notion of 'corporate responsibility' was particularly to the fore as the espoused philosophy of the establishment. This appeared to render a formal co-keyworking scheme irrelevant. Cover was individually negotiated and appeared to be all pervasive. Keyworkers substituted for each other to provide 24 hour cover. Individuals would step into each other's roles in cases of absence.

The Director of Care stated that substitution was made for the role of prime carer when they were not on duty in order to provide 24 hour cover. Records and messages were said to be kept to ensure good communication and continuity. According to the Director the notion of corporate responsibility of the whole staff team was very strong. The Director stated that the dual notion of prime care/ overall responsibility provided the focus of the system. The practice of this may be judged from the notes of the interviews:

A service user interviewed here was not aware of the prime carer system as staff changed three times a day.

> They do a report at the end of the shift . . . . Responsibility is allocated and there is always someone responsible.

A supervisor stated that if the prime carer was off sick other staff may step into the role on overtime.

A service user and their relative both commented that the supervisor and primary carer acted together. 24 hour cover was fine because the director of care was always available.

A primary carer on the night shift said,

> If there is a problem I will phone in or come in during the day e.g. if one of them is not well. One is never off the job and one has a wider responsibility. We cover one another . . . people can be called in and generally help out if they are stuck.

The primary carer who was senior care on the night shift commented that when other primary carers were absent one would tend to check and give cover.

Thus it may be said that this variant of a co-keyworking scheme was based upon corporate notions of team cover rather than upon formal pairing of keyworkers.

3.2 Decision making/meeting needs

A number of common issues in decision making were elaborated by respondents in this establishment these were: a variability in handling longer term planning; the question of rights of service users; and meeting/defining servicing user's needs.

For example, it was said on more than one occasion that the determination of wants when a service user appeared to experience a degree of confusion, and may not be able to make, or communicate their own decision, was said by respondents to be problematic. This appeared generally to be worked through by keyworkers and supervisors via consultation within a network of those concerned including relatives, although assumptions clearly had to be made about service user's views. Practice varied considerably depending upon the quality of the network. The keyworker appeared to have a primary role here in formulating needs and responses. The quality of the relationship between a keyworker and an individual service user was thus of considerable importance in the accuracy (or otherwise) of defining needs.

The Director of Care said:

> In raising individual issues and rights the service user group will tell anyone and will expect things to be acted upon. In informal day to day involvement the prime carer holds a particular role in reflecting service users wants and wishes. Tasks are prioritised in discussion between the prime carer and colleagues and their manager plus the family and service user themselves. The aim is to see things as the service user sees them not as others do (e.g. the GP).

A relative stated that they and the service user were both involved in decisions that affected them. This they said was one of the benefits of having direct contact with the Director of Care (who personally acted as keyworker). Caring was stated by them to be an active process that, for example, involved visits to the theatre, although it was felt that more time could be spent discussing and reminiscing about the past. Time they said was spent over issues such as clothing. The service user was not aware of the prime carer system as staff changed three times a day:

> They do a report at the end of the shift .... Responsibility is allocated and there is always someone responsible. If there is a problem I see the Head of Care and action is taken .... Each day's problems are sorted out. If there is an issue between me and the group, they step in and it's OK .... I am contented as they can talk about things and then things happen .... If I make a point, they take notice and it happens ... (like a bigger wheelchair) .... If there are staff shortages e.g. through sickness then it is noticeable as one may have to get up later that day.

A supervisor who was also primary carer commented that if there was a particular problem the service user would go initially to a member of staff who is on duty. If of particular import it would be relayed to the supervisor/owner on duty. If the prime carer was not able to deal with it in their absence the supervisor may call another member of staff. Similarly if the prime carer was off sick other staff may step into the role on overtime:

> Primary carers can see if service users are having a problem and can talk about it in confidence. They do not take over but go with them. In an individual case they will watch if there is a problem and if not able to deal with it will speak to the Director of Care in order to talk through the issue. Expectations are based upon mutual trust ... Issues tend to be dealt with on a day to day basis rather than through structured meetings. Relationships frame the analysis of needs. The prime carer will need to know all their service users very well and if something is not right pick it up ... [examples here were said to be if they were

unwell or feelings of unease when their family were away on holiday] . . . . The Director of Care meets with each shift and the service users when they wish to join in. This is to decide what is to be done. Other communications may be via the report book. If a service user is not happy with an issue they will say so . . . . In sorting out priorities the prime carer will talk to their supervisor. Flexibility is the keynote. They will try to do what the service user wants. They will deal with what is the most pressing and its significance (e.g. compare minor bleeding with a major fall).

A primary carer on the night shift stated:

> . . . We carry out particular tasks for service users, for example, one resident will only be bathed by their prime carer, if they are away they may not want a bath for four weeks! . . . . A service user will see the primary carer if they are not happy about something. We sort it out and if necessary see the manager on duty . . . . Day to day its via the relationships enabling communication. There is a continual focus on service users on their comfort and well being. We go and see them and if they are OK when we are in . . . . Tasks are prioritised by negotiation with service users e.g. the timing of drinks.

A primary carer who was also housekeeper /laundry assistant stated that issues were brought up by service users with the primary carer or the head of care. The primary carer she said had to deal with this and handle the issue well so as to establish trust:

> . . . It is confidence that establishes the pattern of relationships . . . . Priorities are determined by what one feels has to be done. One aims to keep people in contact and comfortable. It is important to keep conversation so as to get to know them and keep memories alive.

A primary carer (senior care on the night shift) stated that decision making would tend to be done by the manager in consultation with the primary carer. The chain of communication on issues being raised was said by her to be as follows:

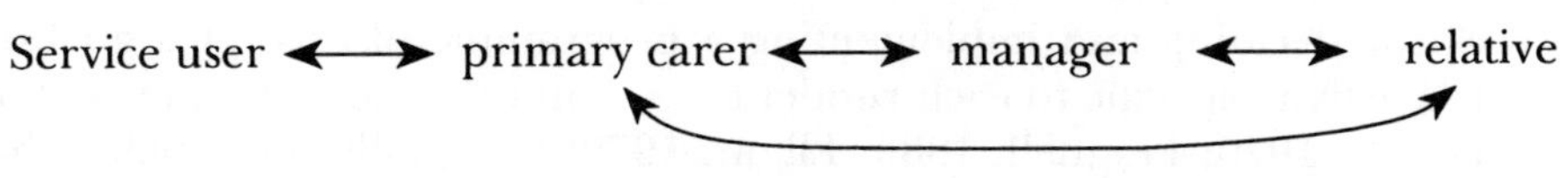

although she said that on an issue such as new clothing the primary carer would tend to deal with the relative direct:

> Primary carers get to know what can be left and what has to take priority. Medical needs are particularly important here and tend to be discussed with the head of care whilst other needs will be discussed with the service user in terms of priority. For example in relation to decision about getting up the service user will dictate direct to the primary carer who in discussion will act on such instructions. By talking to service users the primary carer will get to know their ins and outs the analogy is that by living with them one knows their likes and dislikes.

A relative stated however that there was no forward planning so far as she knew. Any problems or issues were raised by her because of her father's condition. He would raise an issue with her on one of her daily visits and then she raised it with the staff: usually with whoever was in charge at the time. This would depend upon the shift. The staff were said by her to be very helpful and sort problems out:

> . . . The staff tend to assess a problem and therefore whether it should be dealt with as a priority. They may discuss it with me and I may talk to my father about it. If something needs talking through this is done.

The complexity of decision making and accountability was particularly noticeable in this establishment. Day to day decisions in the ethos of care would be taken by the keyworker/ the person on duty who was seen as substitute, or may be referred up the line to the supervisor or to the Director of Care. The tension between decisions in the immediate keyworker/service user relationship and the wider aspects of managerial accountability, would appear to be a primary factor here.

It may be said that as in Burningham (1983) relationships appear here to form a basis aspects of keyworking that concern decision making in meeting needs. Part of this is the question of who makes the rules within relationships and within daily living. Burningham (1983) also discussed the importance of ethos in relation to roles taken by keyworkers. Ethos and role appear to be of considerable importance in this establishment.

Ward's (1978, p 1) suggestion that a keyworker system offers: 'a framework for deciding and implementing a programme of care plus goal directed activity specific to each resident . . . .' and the view of other writers (Sackville, 1979; Pragnell, 1983; Elliott, 1978; and Mallinson, 1989a) that the keyworker is responsible for ensuring that an individual care plan is evolved; updating, implementing, monitoring progress, and conducting reviews; is not entirely borne out in this establishment. The care planning was more fluid than a formalised system. Keyworkers completed checklists which were utilised in occasional reviews . The question explored below under the detailed discussion of needs is how effective the alternative (semi-formal system) actually is.

It may now be said, in relation to this establishment, that:

- informal day to day involvement of service users in decisions was actively pursued by keyworkers.
- keyworkers may prioritise tasks in discussion with senior staff (e.g. in supervision) and by discussion with service users.
- supervision of keyworkers may tend to discuss day to day events, in the context of individual goal – setting and overall plans for the setting.

These aspects of practice are now further explored below in relation to the particular themes comprising this study.

1. Tasks undertaken by keyworkers and how these tasks were prioritised and carried out

In this establishment interviewers indicated that tasks undertaken by keyworkers generally consisted of monitoring, meeting defined needs and undertaking physical care. Tasks were prioritised in discussion with senior staff (e.g. in supervision) and by discussion with service users.

Earlier the Director of Care had indicated in the census questionnaire the list of tasks undertaken by prime carers in order of priority: communication in relationships ('Sitting and listening to residents joys and worries etc.'); Admissions; Assessment of residents; Advocating resident's needs; Physical care; Counselling; Recording; Supporting daily living; Arranging individual outings; and Arranging activities Extreme variability of practice (and what was deemed important or not in relation to needs other than physical care) occurred, however in interpretations of many of the tasks carried out by keyworkers. There were clear differences (in terms of tasks focusing upon a broader range of needs) between managers (as keyworkers) and other staff also acting as keyworkers.

In the process of monitoring, e.g. checking health, most of the recordings in the daily log kept on each service user were completed by keyworkers. These were said by the Director of Care to be 'meaningful recordings'. The prime carer would (according to the Director) review these and discuss them with the service user. Keyworkers filled in check lists upon which they also based discussions with the care manager/supervisor, GP and family to reach informal agreement where there were special needs. Individual keyworkers created a shared view of priorities between service users and themselves. Some short term decisions would then be made on a daily basis.

A primary carer who was on the night shift stated that planning was a day to day thing although reviews were based upon information passed along the line to the supervisor (reports/updating by every member of staff on likes and dislikes). She said that links with relatives were via good rapport. The emphasis was upon making the service user feel happy and assessing what clothes and toiletries were needed or excursions out were required:

> The first point of contact will be made by the primary carer with relatives as they have rights for their parents. The primary carers task is to give them confidence by being happy and cheerful. The managers will also talk to them about needs depending whether an issue is trivial or important . . . . If something is not OK the relatives contact the primary carer and we get it sorted out. I feel they appreciate it. Primary care is like being another relative e.g. going to funerals or buying clothes.

One of the supervisors who also acted as primary carer said:

> Primary carers see relatives on a weekly or daily basis. There are open visiting hours and rotas/matching of prime carers are arranged to the most likely time that relatives are available . . . . If there was a problem the prime carer see the relative specifically to deal with it.

A primary carer on the night shift stated that, in the keyworker role they carried out particular tasks for/with service users e.g.:

> . . . One resident will only be bathed by their prime carer, if they are away they may not want a bath for four weeks! The service user see the primary carer if they are not happy about something. They sort it out and if necessary see the manager on duty . . . . Day to day it's via the relationships enabling communication. There is a continual focus on service users on their comfort and well being. We go and see them and if they are OK when we are in. Tasks are prioritised by negotiation with service users e.g. the timing of drinks.

One primary carer stated that priorities were determined by:

> What one feels has to be done. One aims to keep people in contact and comfortable. It is important to keep (in) conversation so as to get to know them and keep memories alive.

In continuing to focus upon the issue that often what was important was largely entirely individually determined and acted upon, a primary carer (senior care on the night shift) stated that:

> Primary carers get to know what can be left and what as to take priority. Medical needs are particularly important here and tend to be discussed with the head of care whilst other needs will be discussed with the service user in terms of priority. For example in relation to decision about getting up the service user will dictate direct to the primary carer who in discussion will act on such instructions. By talking to service users the primary carer will get to know their ins and outs the analogy is that by living with them one knows their likes and dislikes.

The definition of the role and task of the keyworker and the apparent variability of individual keyworker practice in the determinations of priorities, may be related to the 'good practice theory' of the literature, Meteyard (1986) suggests how roles and tasks for individualisation may be developed and agreed with those involved. This is however based upon an establishment wide interpretation of priorities across the establishment as a whole rather that of individual supervisors. Fulcher and Ainsworth (1985) in describing keyworker responsibilities in group care for children, state that: 'The primary task of a keyworker is to be a special person in the eyes of the child and to be responsible for liaison with others on behalf of that child' (p 230). This again is based upon systems for planning and a clear overall sense of purpose.

It may be argued that the task definition in this keyworker system is too dependent here upon key people such as the Director of Care and individual supervisors many of whom have a different interpretation of priorities.

Following Cambridge (1992) and Dant and Gearing (1990) keyworkers in residential care will assume some direct care support for individual service users. They have the potential to enable service user's day to day needs to be monitored and support to be provided. The detailed knowledge of service users that is necessary for planning may be gained through such daily contact. This is valid in this establishment. The issue is however the degree to which actual practice is dependent upon individuals in the absence of firmly laid down structures and requirements.

2. Networks: Other professionals with whom keyworkers have regular contact.

Generally speaking keyworker networks focused upon the service user's family. Contact with other professionals was rarer and related particularly to medical matters. The involvement of management was likely to happen on all these occasions where decisions were involved, although in day to day matters keyworkers would take the main initiative (e.g. in making relatives feel welcome).

The Director of Care stated that, in the process of monitoring e.g. checking health, prime carers would fill in check lists upon which they based discussions with the care manager/supervisor, GP and family to reach informal agreement where there were special needs. When this stage was reached the Director maintained that all the staff would be advised and the prime carer would co-ordinate and review to make sure that things happen. The keyworker was thus with their supervisor the manager of the care plan, and would (for example) carry out any home assessments. Thus in the process of decision making and defining and meeting needs keyworkers were said to have considerable contact with other persons involved in the process of care.

A service user and their relative commented that their links with the Director of Care (as primary carer) and worked well e.g. if the Doctor had to be called. They were both involved in decisions that affected them. This was said to be one of the benefits of having direct contact with the Director of Care.

One of the supervisors who also acted as primary carer stated:

> Prime carers see relatives on a weekly or daily basis. There are open visiting hours and rotas/matching of prime carers were arranged to the most likely time that relatives were available . . . . If there is a problem the prime carer see the relative specifically to deal with it.

A primary carer stated:

> If something is not OK the relatives contact the primary carer and we get it sorted out. I feel they appreciate it. Primary care is like being another relative e.g. going to funerals or buying clothes.

Another primary carer said:

> Links with relatives are direct by the primary carer to establish trust and enable to become part of the family. In planning to meet needs one seeks the relative's support to establish security for the service user.

A relative commented that they were not involved in care planning. The staff were said to keep on top of issues in meeting service user's needs by their alertness. Accountability he said was an important issues for primary carers. A different relative commented that whilst relatives were involved in terms of information giving and creating an awareness of what was going on, they were not involved in planning. If decisions were required to be made it was suggested that the staff would get on with it but keep relatives informed.

A primary carer who was the senior care on the night shift said that planning tended to be a day to day affair with an emphasis upon making the service user feel happy and assessing what clothes and toiletries were needed or excursions out required:

> The first point of contact will be made by the primary carer with relatives as they have rights for their parents. The primary carers task is to give them confidence by being happy and cheerful. The managers will also talk to them about needs depending whether an issue is trivial or important . . . in raising individual issues and rights the service user group will tell anyone and will expect things to be acted upon. In informal day to day involvement the prime carer holds a particular role in reflecting service users wants and wishes. Tasks are prioritised in discussion between the prime carer and colleagues and their manager plus the family and service user themselves. The aim is to see things as the service user sees them not as others do (e.g. the GP).

A relative stated that they and the service user were both involved in decisions that affected them. This they said was one of the benefits of having direct contact with the Director of Care. Caring was stated by them to be an active process that e.g. involved visits to the theatre, although it was felt that more time could be spent discussing and reminiscing about the past. Time they said was spent over issues such as clothing however.

The primary focus upon the service user's family coupled with occasional contact with medical personnel indicates the isolation (in decision making terms) of keyworker practice in this establishment. The involvement of management where decisions were involved shows the accountability of practice on one hand but also the embryonic nature of professional practitioner keyworker roles on the other. When day to day matters are involved and practitioner keyworkers take the main initiative relationships rather than decision making appear to be the main focus of practice.

In the literature, it was Cambridge (1992) and Dant and Gearing (1990) who maintained that keyworkers in residential care now (in addition to their direct caring role) need to liaise closely with decision makers, feeding information directly into IPP or case reviews, or indirectly via other workers such as case/care managers. This is valid in this establishment, but in practice this appears to be carried out in conjunction with supervisors where decisions of import are involved (as distinct from day to day issues within the relationship). The basis of monitoring by practitioner keyworkers within this establishment is located within structures and on issues determined elsewhere. It is only when the roles of supervisor and keyworker are combined that professional and relationship issues are taken in tandem by the same person.

These processes within networks raise questions of the limitations of the role of keyworkers. That is the theme to be examined next.

3. Limitations of the role of keyworkers

The notion of corporate responsibility was said by the Director of Care to provide the focus of the system in this establishment. In practice this was said to mean that each primary carer had a responsibility for all the group as well as for individuals. The dual notion of prime care/ overall responsibility was said to be very strong.

Individualisation within the corporate approach would in theory place keyworking within the wider context of overall work required in living groups and the residential experience as a whole. One primary carer defined her place in the system as:

> I have a wider responsibility for three small groups but have primary carer responsibility for five of the twenty five service users. I was allocated these five because they had particular needs on the night shift . . . . I do things special [for them] whilst still meeting all the needs [of the residents as a whole].

In reviewing the overall effect of the system, one relative said, 'The more primary carer caring there is the better. Its a good system otherwise staff would not cope. A named individual is very helpful. They are accountable: you know where the buck stops.' Thus the prime carer was said to be responsible to make sure that things happened in their personal practice, particularly after /during the process of care planning. The keyworker with their supervisor was the manager of the care plan. In practice roles were shared, often the supervisor took the lead in decision making and the keyworker the lead in forming direct relationships with service users and relatives in day to day matters. The staff were said to keep on top of issues in meeting service user's needs by their alertness.

Keyworkers were committed in many cases beyond the call of formal conditions of service. One primary carer on the night shift said:

> If there is a problem I will phone in or come in during the day e.g. if one of them is not well. One is never off the job and one has a wider responsibility. We cover one another . . . people can be called in and generally help out [each other] if they are stuck.

These notions of commitment varied between keyworkers. The degree to which they pursued individual issues for their service users also varied. For example, (in contrast to the implications of statements already reported in this section) one relative commented that they were not involved in care planning at all.

For those relatives and service users that knew the system and were able to make their needs known, keyworking /corporate obligations provided a clear sense of who was responsible for an issue and would enable things to happen. One supervisor said:

> 'If there is a particular problem the service user will go initially to a member of staff who is on duty. If [it is] of particular import it would be relayed to the supervisor/ owner on duty. If the prime carer was not able to deal with it in their absence, the supervisor may call another member of staff. Similarly if the prime carer was off sick other staff may step into the role on overtime. . In an individual case they will watch if there is a problem and if not able to deal with it (they) will speak to the Director of Care in order to talk through the issue . . . . The Director of Care meets with each shift and the service users when they wish to join in. This is to decide what is to be done. Other communications may be via the report book. If a service user is not happy with an issue they will say so . . . . In sorting out priorities the prime carer will talk to their supervisor. Flexibility is the keynote. They will try to do what the service user wants. They will deal with what is the most pressing and its significance......'

The role in practice was (according to some primary carers) based upon carrying out particular tasks for service users. Decision making was the province of the manager in consultation with primary carers. A chain of communication/ command was said by one primary carer to be as follows:

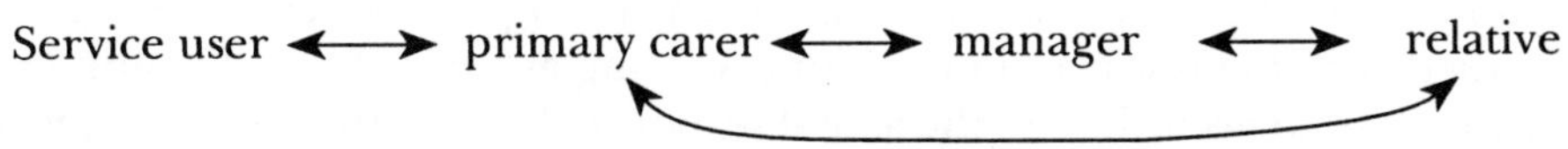

although she said that on an issue such as new clothing the primary carer would tend to deal with the relative direct.

> Primary carers [she said] get to know what can be left and what has to take priority. Medical needs are particularly important here and tend to be discussed with the head of care whilst other needs will be discussed with the service user in terms of priority. For example in relation to decision about getting up the service user will dictate direct to the primary carer who in discussion will act on such instructions. By

talking to service users the primary carer will get to know their ins and outs the analogy is that by living with them one knows their likes and dislikes.

There appears to be here a clear linking of relationships and accountability /responsibility.

The complexity of decision making and accountability was particularly noticeable in this establishment. Day to day decisions in the ethos of care would be taken by the keyworker/ the person on duty who was seen as substitute, or may be referred up the line to the supervisor or to the Director of Care. The tension between decisions in the immediate keyworker/service user relationship and the wider aspects of managerial accountability, would appear to be a primary factor here.

The view in most of the developmental literature is that the role of keyworker is central in care planning (RCA, 1976 and 1983). Implementation, monitoring progress, reviews, records and maintaining relationships are involved here. Howe (1990) suggestion that assessment and management of risk and Fulcher and Ainsworth's (1985) description of a direct care worker co-ordinates all aspects of care and treatment with authority to make decisions, are not entirely borne out in practice here. Many of these roles are the province of the supervisor who works with the keyworker.

The limitations of the definition of role compared with the theory of keyworking raises the issue of what authority a keyworker has and how this affects their responsibility and accountability. That theme we will examine next.

4. Authority, responsibility and accountability of keyworkers

Accountability of keyworkers occurred within the network of care. Responsibilities and the authority to act were defined within the supervisory relationship. Extreme variability of practice occurred between different keyworkers. There were also clear difference between managers (as keyworkers) who merged both the roles, and practitioners acting as keyworkers. Accountability thus varied according to the actual responsibility and the authority given to individual keyworkers to act.

In the complexity of decision making and accountability day to day decisions in the ethos of care would be taken by the keyworker/ the person on duty who was seen as substitute, or may be referred up the line to the supervisor or to the Director of Care. The tension between decisions in the immediate keyworker/service user relationship and the wider aspects of managerial accountability, would appear to be a primary factor here. Some illustrations of the variability of the way practice was framed are given so that the effect of this may be assessed.

One service user homed in on the corporate notion of responsibility rather than keyworkers being particularly responsible for individualising care:

> Responsibility is allocated and there is always someone responsible . . . . If there is a problem I see the Head of Care and action is taken.'

In contrast, a relative said,

> The more primary carer caring there is the better. Its a good system otherwise staff would not cope. A named individual is very helpful. They are accountable: you know where the buck stops.

A relative reinforced this notion of accountability to persons with a defined interest in the process and outcomes of care:

> If decisions are required to be made the staff will get on with it but keep relatives informed.'

Overall the impression generated within the interviews is one of service users and relatives needing to be clear on an individual basis how particular variations in the system affected them. These variations were there for good reason, e.g. how capable a particular keyworker was and what it was appropriate for them to carry out given their degree of competence. Variations in responsibility given to individual keyworkers were a strength of the system but also a weakness. Accountability was thus dependent upon what duties were prescribed and therefore focused mainly upon the managerial hierarchy. This resulted in authority also being managerially prescribed rather than reflecting service user power and choice within the keyworker relationship.

Many of these issues reflect the views of Davis (1978) who highlighted ambiguities in keyworking practice. He specifically mentions 'the shadow of accountability [and] divided loyalties' in the context of confidentiality, communication, and power in/ the power of relationships. He identified the structural problem of an employee who is expected to be accountable to both service user and manager. In the notion of corporate responsibility the primary focus here, in this establishment, is on meeting service user need. Managerial based accountability is shared accountability where there is a sense of the paying customer in the private sector. Non-the less the keyworker can only be as good as other workers and the system allow. The ethos of the establishment dictates the dynamics of where primary accountability lies and what its effect actually is.

These issues set the scene for a discussion of the next theme concerning the process of meeting needs of service users.

The process of care planning has already been reported upon in this chapter in relation to tasks undertaken by keyworkers. The system espoused by the Director of Care involved the prime carer taking the initial role in recording and checking on needs, reviewing these and discussing these with the service user and then with the care manager/supervisor, GP and family to reach informal agreement on requirements. This particularly applied where special needs were involved. All staff were, said to then be advised by the primary carer of the goals involved. The prime carer would co-ordinate and review progress making sure that the goals were achieved. The keyworker was thus said to be the manager of the care plan, and would (for example) carry out any home assessments.

In practice much of these roles were carried out by the supervisor although in informal day to day involvement the prime carer held a particular role in advocating service users wants and wishes. Where supervisors were also primary carers the roles were combined and this appeared to work well. There was also a wide variation in roles and in practices depending upon the ability of the keyworker and how they were managed by individual supervisors.

Some relatives were involved in planning others not. For some service users meeting needs was said by their primary carer to be 'largely a day to day affair with an emphasis upon making the service user feel happy and assessing what clothes and toiletries were needed or excursions out required.' For others it involved a good deal of planning and networking.

Keyworkers commented that small group provision helped to focus on meeting day to day needs as differences were particularly apparent in the context of the service user/keyworker relationship. A shared view of these was said to be obtained.

The determination of wants when a service user appeared to experience a degree of confusion and may not be able to make or communicate their own decision may also be seen on occasions as problematic. This issue appeared to be worked through in this establishment by consultation within a network of those concerned including relatives, although assumptions may clearly have to be made about service user's views. The keyworker appeared to have a primary role in this respect. The quality of the relationship between a keyworker and an individual service user was of considerable importance here.

Needs of service users were officially placed on the planning agenda within the management structure based upon the keyworker acting as initial advocate drawing it to the supervisors attention. As one primary carer said:

> Primary carers can see if service users are having a problem and can talk about it in confidence. They do not take over but go with them. In

an individual case they will watch if there is a problem and if not able to deal with it will speak to the Director of Care in order to talk through the issue. Expectations are based upon mutual trust . . . . Relationships frame the analysis of needs. The prime carer will need to know all their service users very well and if something is not right pick it up . . . . In sorting out priorities the prime carer will talk to their supervisor . . . . They will try to do what the service user wants.

Another Primary carer pointed out discussions with service users concerning a hierarchy of needs, priorities and action:

> Medical needs are particularly important . . . and tend to be discussed with the head of care whilst other needs will be discussed with the service user in terms of priority. For example in relation to decision about getting up the service user will dictate direct to the primary carer who in discussion will act on such instructions. By talking to service users the primary carer will get to know their . . . likes and dislikes.

Relatives were involved in defining needs. One stated that issues would be raised by them with the primary carer on visits or with whoever was in charge at the time depending upon the shift:

> The staff tend to assess a problem and therefore whether it should be dealt with as a priority. They may discuss it with me and I may talk to my father about it. If something needs talking through this is done.

Inputs appeared to vary according to the particular keyworker and the relationship they may have with the service user (and relatives). Thus the amount that they are 'part of the service user's life space' varied. The actual defining of the nature of the life space generally appeared to be a variety of people other then the service user themselves although there were a few notable exceptions.

The question of who makes the rules concerning defining needs within relationships and within daily living (Burningham 1983) is clearly of importance here. Ward (1978, p 1) suggestion that a keyworker system offers: 'a framework for deciding and implementing a programme of care plus goal directed activity specific to each resident' is probably true but of variable effect depending upon the systems and structures involved. This variable dependency upon systems and the way they operate would also apply to the principles espoused by other writers such as Sackville (1979), Mallinson (1989a), Pragnell (1983), and Elliott (1978).

Certainly the view that occurs throughout the literature that the role of keyworker is central in care planning processes (For example, RCA 1976 and 1983) is confirmed. Keyworkers in this establishment either process care planning or act to draw issues into the care planning agenda.

The dangers expressed by Davis (1978) whereby the keyworker may be incorporated into a 'spurious consensus' with other professional colleagues at the expense of the weakest party – the service user – was one that it may be maintained was only alleviated here by good management. Some keyworkers had however clearly here, as in the practice Davis reports, developed relationships with service users of such quality that they became totally available and involved as advocates for service user's rights and champions in individualised development. As a decision maker, a keyworker may only be as good as other workers and the system allow.

SCA's (1988) attempts to locate keyworking within the wider framework for the delivery of care may be suggested to be a necessary requirement. Keyworking is only part of wider structures within which to implement principles, and objectives.

4. Summary: effect of this keyworker system

By way of a summary a number of factors may be stated in relation to the effect of this keyworker system:

1. Individualised care

- Short term decisions occurred on a daily basis.
- Keyworkers monitored service users on health matters through check lists upon which they subsequently discussed with the care manager/ supervisor, GP and family to reach informal agreement where there were special needs.
- The keyworker in conjunction with their supervisor was the manager of the service user's care plan.
- In informal day to day involvement the keyworker held a particular role in reflecting service users wants and wishes.
- Service users and their relatives commented that they were involved in decisions that affected them.
- Planning was a day to day thing although reviews were based upon information passed along the line to the supervisor
- The support of relatives was sought in care planning to meet needs and to establish a sense of security for the service user
- There was no direct evidence that care planning by keyworkers assisted in enabling them to promote shared decision or making and service user choice
- Informal day to day involvement of service users in decisions is actively pursued by keyworkers.

- Keyworkers prioritise tasks in discussion with senior staff (e.g. in supervision) and by discussion with service users.
- In informal day to day involvement the keyworker held a particular role in reflecting service users wants and wishes.

2. Relationships

- Keyworking was based upon developing relationships.
- Matching was by personalities but within small group living units, based upon creatively developing relationships. The service user had the choice of the person they got on well with.
- A creative view of the task of the keyworker was taken that was linked to small group living.
- Keyworkers often saw relatives on a weekly or daily basis.
- Rotas/matching of keyworkers were arranged to the most likely time that relatives were available.
- Expectations were said by keyworkers to be based upon mutual trust
- Relationships framed the analysis of needs.

3. Clarity of the residential task

- The notion of corporate responsibility of the whole staff team was strong. The dual notion of keyworking/ overall responsibility provided the focus of the system.
- Variability in the involvement of relatives by keyworkers occurred.
- The difference between the practice of managers (as keyworkers) and other staff also acting as keyworkers appeared marked.
- Keyworkers were said by relatives to be accountable: 'you know where the buck stops'.
- Variations in practice in care planing occurred in relation to links into every day decisions and the sense of accountability of keyworkers.
- supervision of keyworkers tends to discuss day to day events, in the context of individual goal – setting and overall plans for the setting.
- Tasks are prioritised in discussion between the keyworker and colleagues and their manager plus the family and service user.
- decision making tended to be done by the manager in consultation with the keyworker.
- A chain of communication existed as follows:

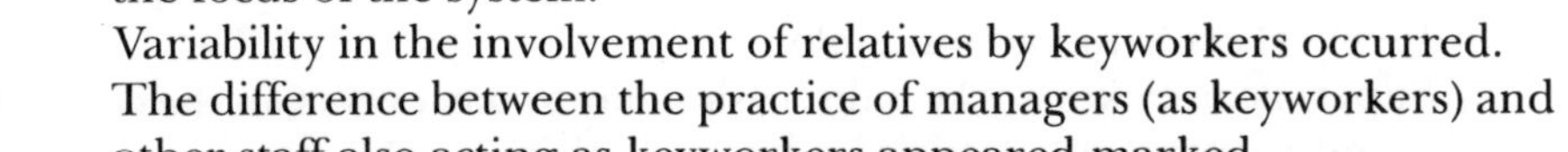

- There appeared to be here a clear linking of relationships and accountability/responsibility.
- Day to day decisions would be taken by the keyworker/ the person on duty, or may be referred up the line.

5. Conclusions

The particular strengths of this keyworker system in contributing towards improved individualised care may be said to involve:

- Keyworkers monitoring special needs through the structure of check lists discussing these with those involved.
- The keyworker role of reflecting service users wants and wishes.
- Involvement of service users and their relatives in decisions that affected them.
- The support of relatives sought in care planning to establish a sense of security for the service user.
- A creative view of the keyworker task linked to small group living.
- Rotas/matching of keyworkers arranged to the most likely time that relatives were available.
- Relationships framing the analysis of needs.
- The dual notion of prime care/ overall responsibility providing the focus of the system.
- Keyworkers being accountable.
- Supervision of keyworkers discussing day to day events, in the context of individual goal – setting and overall plans for the setting.
- A clear chain of communication.
- A linking of relationships and accountability/responsibility.
- The focus in care planning upon individual day to day needs and practice.
- Small group provision linking meeting needs to the keyworker role.
- Consultation on defining needs taking place within a network of those concerned, including relatives.
- Analysis of needs framed within relationships.
- Informal day to day involvement of service users in decisions being actively pursued by keyworkers.
- Keyworkers prioritising tasks in discussion with senior staff (e.g. in supervision) and in discussion with service users.
- Responsibility being allocated and there being always someone responsible.
- A named individual that was accountable.
- Expectations based upon mutual trust.
- Relationships linked with accountability and responsibility.

The weaknesses of this particular keyworker system in terms of its ability to contribute towards improved individualised care may be said to involve:

- Variability in the involvement of relatives by keyworkers.
- Differences between the practice of managers (as keyworkers) and other staff also acting as keyworkers.
- Variations in practice in care planing in relation to links into every day decisions and the sense of accountability of keyworkers.

As was the case in the statutory sector establishment, the overall impression that appears to pertain here is a variability in the nature and quality of practice within many of the dimensions explored. The question may be asked again whether these are strengths and weaknesses of keyworker systems in general, or only of this particular keyworker system. In a further endeavour to answer this question, comparisons may be made between this and the statutory sector establishment. The next chapter considers this and in a move beyond evaluating individual strengths and weaknesses attempts to draw some overall conclusions relative to the central issue of this book: Whether keyworking in residential care for older people contributes towards improved individualised care.

7 Implications of differing systems and practices: Recommendations for policy, strategy, organisation and practice

1. Introduction

The quality of practice in these keyworker systems appears to be generally dependent upon variations within other structures (such as those for supervision, evaluation and for care planning) and upon the variable nature of practice carried out by individual keyworkers in individualising care. The effect of the quality and particular style of management in each of the establishments, and in the ethos, appears to also have a significant effect upon differences in the practice of keyworkers in individualising care.

This chapter compares keyworking in the two case study establishments (previously discussed individually in chapters 5 and 6). From these comparisons the implications of the strengths and weaknesses of practice are analysed, and recommendations are made. A set of principles for sound practice in the areas of relationships, decision making and the role of keyworkers are generated, based upon the findings of this book. These together with the wider recommendations for practice will form a basis from which to tackle the major weaknesses of keyworker systems and to build upon the strengths of systems in order to firmly establish keyworker systems of quality reflecting the requirements of the late 1990s.

Finally the central question posed within this book: Does keyworking in residential care for older people contribute towards improved individualised care? is examined and some conclusions are reached. The recommendations and principles for practice development proposed herein may then be seen in the context of what keyworker systems have to offer to improving practice in individualising care.

2.1 Findings: (a) The strengths of keyworker systems in creating purposeful relationships for individualising care within group living

As we saw in chapters 5 and 6 there were felt to be a number of strengths within keyworking. These were formulated as a result of exploring practice themes suggested by the research agenda within the two establishments concerned. The strengths of the keyworking approach appear to lie in the application of individualisation within small group experiences, and in creating a sense of focus beyond physical care to meet emotional needs. Planning to meet a broader range of needs appears to be able to be facilitated readily within keyworking practice. These strengths tally with the bulk of the literature on keyworking (e.g. Rodway, 1981; Burningham, 1983; and Hopkins et al, 1984).

Burningham (1983) and Rodway (1981) saw the special relationship with service users build up as a result of keyworkers carrying out the task of individualising care in ways that emphasised companionship and sharing. The sense of focus here may now be said to be particularly realised where the quality of service and action taken by the individual keyworker is the primary agenda. In the context of group interaction, Hopkins et al. (1984) extended these arguments by highlighting shared expectations created within the relationship.

The particular forms of relationships that are associated with keyworker practice appear (where individual practice, other structures and systems permit) to be able to promote the quality of life within residential care. Keyworking appears to be a benefit to service users in situations where structures, and systems allow the benefits of individualised practice to come to the fore. It is clear that keyworking can promote clarity in the nature of the task carried out by the worker, accountability and job satisfaction.

Individual themes are discussed below in relation to the two case study establishments:

1. Nature of keyworker/service user relationships

There were differences between the two establishments in the way relationships focus upon the nature of the task. These are summarised in Table 10.1.

These differences were derivative of the style and ethos of the establishments as a whole. The aims of keyworking were generally set by the guidelines produced by management. This is indicative of a variability in keyworker systems, a perceived flexibility in the ability of different systems to meet different situations. It could however also be construed as a weakness in not having a common formulation. The common ground between the two establishments lies in the general focus upon providing a service to residents through the keyworker relationship.

Table 7.1
Comparison of nature of keyworker and service user relationships

	Large statutory establishment	Small private establishment
Nature/focus of Relationship		1. Developing trust
	2. Personalised care	
	3. Responsive service	3. Service provided as recipients require
		4. To make the home a happy place and service users content

Overall it appears that purposeful relationships can be built up and reciprocated. Effective relationships were said to focus upon mutual trust. Reciprocation and trust was said to often be established when there was a clear sense of purpose within the context of individualising care. The keyworker role appeared to be effective when focusing upon meeting needs. In establishing this sense of focus, Keyworkers and the service users worked together on requirements and decisions.

These findings may now be allied with the views of Burningham (1983), Hopkins et al. (1984), and Rodway (1981) already reported in this chapter. Their views express a prescription for effective keyworking practice whereby keyworkers may create unique and special relationships with service users that build upon individualising care, focusing upon giving a service of quality of service defined by shared expectations formulated within the relationship.

Arising out of this discussion it is recommended that:

- Clear aims and a sense of purpose are framed to provide a base for the practice of individual keyworkers. The linking of keyworker systems to the ethos of the establishment be carried out by design and the nature of the keyworker task set out in documents of guidance.

- Relationships between keyworkers and service users be built up carefully over a period, establishing firmly a sense of mutual trust.

- Keyworkers see their role as particularly focusing upon meeting needs, working together with service users on requirements and decisions.

- Keyworkers strive to build/ achieve effective relationships with a clear sense of purpose focusing upon meeting needs within the context of jointly agreed decisions.

2. Relationship between keyworking and small living groups

Keyworking appeared to be effective in enabling the framing of individual needs. This often took place in both establishments within the group context and in small living units. This focus upon the group as well as the individual appears to addresses the possible weakness highlighted in the theoretical exploration of the literature on residential care by Elkan and Kelly (1991) Individualised care is taken here in the context of the group experience rather than merely creating an individualised response to the provision of services. Every day care was also a team function but one based upon the keyworkers input. Keyworkers in building relationships also enabled group interaction. A creative view of the keyworker task in meeting needs linked to interaction within small group living appeared to provide the best practice formula. Relationships that linked with accountability and responsibility in providing individualised care appeared to enable a clear sense of purpose.

This linking with the wider framework of caring reinforces the contemporary suggestions of SCA (1988, and 1991) The formula in the 1988 document locates keyworking firmly within the wider framework for the delivery of care and includes wider interactions and teamwork. The management of keyworking systems is said by SCA to be central to creating these links. The 1991 document formalises this by systematically considering the integration of individualised care, teamwork, relationships, care planning and supervision.

Whilst there were a number of differences between the two establishments, there were also many similarities that could be drawn out in assessing the relationship of keyworking to small living groups. These similarities and differences are summarised in Table 10.2.

The additional points contained in the table, in relation to the large statutory establishment may be explained by the nature and size of the building and therefore the actual nature of the group living experience. Overall it may be said that in both establishments keyworking and small group living are dynamically linked particularly in relation to meeting needs.

The SCA documents (1988; and 1991) already mentioned in this section of this chapter, begin to systematically consider the integration of individualised care, teamwork, relationships, in group contexts and may thus provide a secure platform for the development of keyworker systems.

Arising out of this discussion it is recommended that:

Table 7.2
Comparison of relationship between keyworking and small living groups

	Large statutory establishment	Small private establishment
Relationship of keyworking to small group living	1. Unitisation provides focus for particular needs (e.g. dementia). Keyworker allocation follows i.e. semi specialist allocation matching skills to needs.	1. Creative view of task independent of small living groups (interlinked lounges graded by dependency)
	2 Focus for keyworker input.	2. Creates sense of focus and enables staff to work with small number of service users
	3. Enabling communal decision-making	3. Group dominates daily living
	4. Helps communication and localising relationships.	4. Some service users isolate themselves from the group
	5. Keyworkers carry out group tasks but in quieter times of day carry out individualised care e.g. toileting after breakfast	5. Some primary carers have responsibility for group, others a more diffuse spread
	6. Focus for keyworker decision making between individual and group	6. Where applicable (see 5 above) tend to concentrate efforts
	7. Quality of caring said to be more dependent on keyworking than small groups	
	8. Breaks institutional effect: 'makes more manageable'	
	9. Resolve tensions in group living via consultative intervention (ix)	
	10. Group enables relationships outside keyworker system	

- Keyworkers focus upon individualised care within the overall situation of social groups. The linking of individualised care and group living is seen as the primary dynamic of keyworker activities.

- Individual needs are be provided through a named individual in the context of the staff team as a whole. The interrelationship of the staff group and the individual keyworker is developed by managerial strategies promoting team development and individual support.

- Provision for meeting individual needs as co-ordinated by keyworkers is considered within the context of meeting broad needs in the group living situation.

- Individual provision by keyworkers is located in the interactions and decision making that takes place within living groups as well as in the confidential and private context of individual meetings, and the process of individualised caring.

- Keyworkers in building individual relationships should also enable group interaction.

- Relationships are linked with accountability and responsibility in providing individualised care creating a clear sense of purpose.

2.2 Findings: (b) the strengths of keyworker systems in decision making/ meeting needs in individualising care

Exploration of strengths within keyworking practice is continued based upon the themes suggested by the research agenda created in relation to the two case study establishments:

1. Tasks undertaken by keyworkers

There tended to be more differences between the two establishments than similarities in relation to the main tasks of keyworkers. These differences were located in the team context, i.e. they appeared to relate to what were defined as a team responsibility, and what constituted the individualised agenda of keyworkers. The similarities and differences are summarised in Table 10.3.

Generally, the keyworker role, when focused upon care planning, appeared to give a firm sense of structure. Linking relationships with meeting needs (defined through joint decision making) enabled this. A shared view of priorities between service users and keyworkers could occur. Keyworkers

Table 7.3
Comparison of main keyworker tasks

	Large statutory establishment	Small private establishment
Main Keyworker Tasks	1. Bathing	
	2 Purchasing e.g. toiletries	
	3. Produce reports for review meetings	
	4. Attend to practical necessitates e.g. teeth, hearing aids + glasses	
	5. Help user re needs e.g. to cope with dentist	
	6. Prioritise work and determine ways of working e.g. how to feed a particular service user	6. Prioritise by negotiation with service user e.g. timing of drinks
	7. Those 'needed' by and done with service user (e.g. 'clean out wardrobe')	7. Carry out particular tasks for service user with their agreement
	8. Involve relatives in reviews	
		9. To share in service user's life space: read talk and listen, share interests
		10 Encourage activities

undertaking purposeful roles monitored special needs in a structured way discussing these with service users, relatives and other professionals as appropriate. Informal day to day involvement of service users in decisions was actively pursued by keyworkers effective in their role. Keyworkers would prioritise tasks in discussion with senior staff (e.g. in supervision) and in discussion with service users.

The differences between the two establishments may be considered in the context of the position of Douglas and Payne (1987) and Meteyard (1986?) whereby each unit will tends to develop its own prescription of roles and tasks and these may be agreed with those involved.

The focus here upon care planning accords with that of Ward (1978) and RCA (1983) whereby the main role of the keyworker is said to involve individualised care planning, implementation, monitoring progress, reviews, records and maintaining relationships. Monitoring and supporting roles in the process of meeting needs indicates that the potential expressed by Cambridge (1992) and Dant and Gearing (1990) is perfectly practicable to realise. Thus in the context of care planning keyworkers may enable service user's day to day needs to be monitored and support to be provided. The degree to which keyworkers and service users may be involved in formal decision making would appear however to be variable.

It is recommended that:

- The role of the keyworker is focused upon care planning, linking relationships with meeting needs.

- Joint decision making involving service users takes place on a daily basis with a shared view of priorities. This is seen as the norm in keyworker practice.

- A general view of tasks involved in carrying out the role and a sense of priorities is achieved in discussion with senior staff (e.g. in supervision) and in discussion with service users.

2. Networks: other professionals with whom keyworkers have regular contact

Successful links were often made with relatives by keyworkers in both establishments in order to define needs and implement the individual service user's care plan. Part of the task here was the involvement of service users and their relatives in decisions that affected them. The support of relatives sought in care planning appeared to establish a sense of security for the service user. In order to facilitate this contact, rotas/matching of keyworkers could be arranged to meet the most likely time that relatives were available.

This potential of the keyworker as the contact point with relatives and other professionals in the care process has been known for some time, but has tended to be very neglected in the literature. For example, Ward (1978) some years back, discussed the underplaying of the ideal of a keyworker as the person who was responsible for the 'progress through' (pre-admission, admission, and later, discharge and after care) of a service user within the residential experience. There appears, at the time of writing, to be no current conceptualisation in the literature, of the keyworker as the contact point for relatives. Contemporary writings e.g. Cambridge (1992) and Dant and Gearing (1990) suggest an alternative focus, i.e. that keyworkers need to liaise closely with decision makers, feeding information directly into IPP or case reviews, or indirectly via other workers such as case/care managers.

The basis of networking by keyworkers in each establishment is summarised in Table 10.4.

Table 7.4
Comparison of networks maintained by keyworkers

	Large statutory establishment	Small private establishment
Contacts maintained by keyworkers	1. Field Social Workers (where applicable)	
	2. Family network (e.g. in relation to reviews)	2. Family: on weekly basis to deal with problems + obtain agreement on special needs
	3. Medical personnel e.g. GP usually through supervisor	3. Medical personnel e.g. GP usually through supervisor

The keyworker now may be seen as the contact point for professionals, service users and relatives. The individualisation of the care task, it may be suggested, necessitates an individual reference points for all these contacts and a focus here upon meeting needs in the context of care planning.

It is recommended that:

- Keyworkers should be seen as the primary point of contact with relatives. The tasks involved should be facilitated by adjustments of rotas etc.
- Links with relatives by keyworkers are used to define needs and implement the individual service user's care plan. Service users and their relatives are involved, a matter of course, in decisions that affect them.
- The keyworker should be seen as the reference point for contact in relation to care planning by all personnel involved.

3. Limitations of the role of keyworkers

Supervision of keyworkers was used successfully to promote sound practice in day to day events, in the context of individual goal - setting and overall plans for the setting. A clear chain of communication here enabled decision making and formulation of clear boundaries of responsibility.

The tasks undertaken by keyworkers in both establishments derived from the role that it was seen appropriate for them to carry out. This varied between the two establishments depending upon what duties were seen as the responsibility of the keyworkers and what the responsibility of others (members of the team, or the supervisor.) The similarities and differences are summarised in Table 10.5.

These variations appear to accord with the practice formulations of SCA/BASW (1987); SCA (1988); and SCA (1991) whereby respective roles may be divided by agreement between keyworkers and their supervisors. These documents all make the point that these variations are only workable if there is a clarity in their formulation, and if they are subject to review (particularly if there variations exist between role boundaries for different individual workers).

It is recommended that:

- Within supervision sound practice in individual goal - setting in the context of overall plans for the setting is promoted. Day to day events are evaluated particularly how these relate to goal definition and achievement.

- Within supervision agreement should be reached on the nature of the respective roles to be carried out by both keyworkers and supervisors, and upon frameworks for decision making.

4. Authority, responsibility and accountability of keyworkers

Clarity in responsibility and accountability of keyworkers was generally found helpful in both establishments particularly if this reflected service users wants and wishes. The dual notion of keyworking and an overall responsibility appeared to provide a sense of focus to keyworker systems in relation to the broader task in hand. Relationships that linked with accountability provided a firm sense of task for the work of a named individual responsible for providing individualised care.

The areas of accountability of keyworkers in the two establishments were similar in orientation. These are summarised in Table 10.6.

Deciding upon the respective roles of keyworkers and their supervisors by agreement (SCA/BASW, 1987; SCA, 1988; and SCA, 1991) may again be highlighted as relevant.

Table 7.5
Comparison of main keyworker roles

	Large statutory establishment	Small private establishment
Keyworker Roles	1. Decision making ('where above the norm')	1. Discuss issues with service user
	2. Assessment: pre-admission visits + recommendations	2. Make 'meaningful recordings' carry out assessments
	3. Care planning: keyworking said to be fundamental to implementation	3. Manager of care plan with supervisor. Coordinate and review to make things happen
	4. Undertake extra responsibility	
	5. Decide individual special needs on ad hoc basis (fitting in with rotas and other group needs)	
	6. Initial hearer of complaints then take 'appropriate action'	6. To see service user if not happy re something
		7. Attend to basic necessitates
	8. Delegated attention to 'problem areas'	8. To see if service user has problem and talk about it in confidence
	9. In some cases substitute relative	
	10. Filter in hierarchy re 'what is important or not'	
	11. Involvement of service user e.g. in social activities	11. Organise outings
	12. Talk through issues with relatives e.g. if they are upset and get to know the finer points of service users likes and dislikes	12. To always welcome family members and make them feel at home.
		13. Prioritise tasks in discussion with colleagues manager, user and family
		14. Involve family, look after user as if member of family

Table 7.6
Comparison of basis of keyworkers' accountability

	Large statutory establishment	Small private establishment
Accountability of Keyworkers	1. Care staff on each unit informally supervised by the head of each unit who is of officer status	1. All staff no matter what their position (i.e. management, housekeeping, care staff etc.) as keyworkers are supervised informally (as appropriate) by Director of Care or other Management Team member
	2. Informal accountability to relatives	2. Informal accountability to service users in some cases and to relatives via management in all cases

It is recommended that:

- Supervision should be utilised in keyworker systems to promote accountability and decision making. A clear chain of communication will enable decision making and formulation of clear boundaries of responsibility.

5. The way needs of service users are met

Relationships framing the analysis of needs appeared to create a sense of purpose in both establishments. The keyworker role of reflecting service users wants and wishes obtained a greater sense of focus through care planning. Individual day to day needs and practice could be seen in this context. The Keyworker role of monitoring special needs could be carried out through the structured use of items such as check lists discussing these with those involved. Consultation on defining needs should take place within a network of those concerned, including relatives. Analysis of needs were successfully framed within relationships.

This suggestion of the overall context of keyworking being the main focus in the establishment for care planning, defining and meeting needs and individual decision making in daily living is one occurring throughout the keyworker literature (e.g: Ward, 1987; Sackville, 1979; Pragnell, 1983 and Mallinson, 1989a. Plus in relation to networking and liaison: Cambridge, 1992 and Dant and Gearing, 1990).

The practice of the two establishments was similar and is summarised in Table 10.7.

Table 7.7
Comparison of processes undertaken by keyworkers in meeting needs

	Large statutory establishment	Small private establishment
Process of keyworking in meeting needs	1. Joint work keyworker and supervisor to interpret service user's wishes 2. Keyworking fundamental to assessment and to 'get beyond concentration on physical care'	1. Needs examined with supervisor and with Director of Care to decide what is to be done 2. Tends to be day to day discussion

It is recommended that:

- Relationships provide a foundation for care planning within keyworker systems to create purposeful ways of defining and meeting needs. Priorities be defined with the service user and the keyworker role seen as focusing upon monitoring and progressing decision making.

2.3. Findings: (c) the variability of practice: a major weakness of keyworker systems

A number of issues may be drawn out of the common ground between the case studies. These pose fundamental questions within keyworker practice and are:

- The power of the keyworker in decision making and its differential exercise.

- The variable nature of the relationship between keyworker and service user.
- The 'interpretation' of service user's wishes by keyworker and/or supervisor.
- The role of keyworkers in terms of a 'right to intervene' in group living.
- Different philosophies of individual keyworkers and styles of working.
- Quality of supervision in picking up individual differences in practice.
- The comparative quality of practice of individual Keyworkers as a point of first contact in a chain of command.

These conspire to provide the basis for fundamental differences in quality of practice, and interpretation of practice requirements by individual keyworkers and their supervisors. This is an issue that should be tackled if any keyworker system is to be fully effective.

The only literature that hints at problems like these is Davis (1978) and Mallinson and Best (1987) in these articles the issues of power, differential practices by different keyworkers, and collusion by supervisors, were examined. These issues raise fundamental questions concerning the nature of the variability in quality of practice within and between different keyworker systems, and in practice conducted by individual keyworkers and their supervisors.

The preceding section highlighted the variability between different keyworking establishments. Variations depend upon interpretation of the aims of keyworking and the methodology for achieving them. Keyworker systems also appeared to be heavily dependent in structural terms upon the nature and quality of allied systems structures and methodological principles such as those for care planning. These appear to govern the actions of keyworkers and how they interpret/ carry out their role. In turn the way a keyworker system is managed, and the degree to which key personnel such as supervisors take a proactive role, will determine how keyworkers interpret their task and how much they focus upon particular issues within that role.

The quality of practice and issues/ action taken in areas such as relationships, authority, responsibility and accountability also appears to be determined by the nature of the system and how it is managed.

In theory, it is a strength of the keyworker formula, that it countenances flexibility in delivery between different establishments and their philosophies. The danger of this may be however that keyworking can become dilute and meaningless as a conceptual way of working. In some situations it may merely become an empty title; in others it may represent a way of creating purposeful and clear practice, focusing upon delivering quality individualised care within the context of meeting group needs.

At a micro level, within a each separate system and the way it was defined, extreme variability between practice of individual keyworkers occurred in both these establishments. In view of the fact that this then affected the process and outcomes of individualised care this may now be highlighted a major weakness of keyworker systems as presently formulated. This problem occurred as a primary weakness in both establishments. (See, conclusions, chapters 5 and 6). The reasons for this variability of practice appeared to occur mainly because of a lack of consensus regarding: the role of the keyworker, the requirements in fulfilling it and the outcomes required of the supervisory system. In theory, these deficiencies are weaknesses of keyworker systems that can be remedied if action is taken in all these areas; it is not a fatal flaw.

The 'system' appeared in both cases to allow variability by not prescribing minimum requirements and common ways of working between different keyworkers. This was compounded in both establishments by the different capabilities of staff not being addressed. The results then evolved overall into a case of 'do what you feel able to'. The only way the two establishments managed to give a minimum level of service was by a flexible boundary in the definition of responsibilities, between individual keyworkers and their supervisors. The lottery of who was a keyworker (and what they did/ were prepared to do/ the quality of the relationship) gave different levels of service in relation to client choice, participation in decision making and the degree to which care was individualised.

Clearly if decisions were made by managers (acting as keyworkers or on behalf of keyworkers) these had a different sense of authority than ones made by keyworkers themselves. The sense of who was responsible had a variability about it, and thus, who was accountable (and for what) varied. The fact that these issues appeared in variable quantities/ degrees between the two establishments (one having a much larger number of weaknesses in these areas that the other) suggests that these are issues that can be worked through, rather than their being a fatal flaw in the principle of individualised care through named individuals. This can perhaps be done through the way managers work with staff to define, implement, monitor and focus systems. The question of effectiveness of companion structures such as care planning, and supervision and how they impinge / are utilised within keyworker systems in order to work through these weaknesses is an important issue.

It is recommended that:

- The role of the keyworker is clearly defined in all keyworker systems, the minimum requirements in fulfilling the role and common standards should be agreed in the staff team and systems /frameworks set up to ensure that these requirements and standards are met by all concerned.

- The role and outcomes required in supervising keyworkers/ how these are to be achieved be agreed by all concerned. Decision making and monitoring of the effectiveness of the system be initially conducted in such forums as well as within the every day practice of the team.

- Managers define, implement, monitor and focus systems to achieve effectiveness within companion structures such as those for care planning. These structures will need to articulate clearly with keyworking and the roles undertaken by all players within keyworker systems.

Framed by the import of these findings the discussion in the previous chapters may now be translated into principles for promoting sound practice that builds upon strengths and addresses weaknesses in different areas of keyworker operation.

3.1. Developing keyworker practice: practice principles: (a) relationships

This section builds upon the strengths of the keyworking approach. Earlier in this chapter, in the context of relationships these strengths were said to lie in the application of individualisation within small group experiences, and in creating a sense of focus beyond physical care to meet emotional needs. These strengths tally with the bulk of the literature on keyworking (see particularly Rodway, 1981; Burningham, 1983; and Hopkins et al, 1984.) Purposeful relationships can be built up and reciprocated. Effective relationships focus upon mutual trust. Reciprocation and trust are established when there is a clear sense of purpose within the context of individualising care.

The keyworker role is effective when focusing upon meeting needs. In establishing this sense of focus, Keyworkers and the service users work together on requirements and decisions. Keyworking appears to be effective in enabling the framing of individual needs. This often takes place within the group context and in small living units. Individualised care is framed in the context of the group experience rather than merely creating an individualised response to the provision of services. Every day care is also a team function but one based upon the keyworkers input. Keyworkers in building relationships enable group interaction. A creative view of the keyworker task links interaction within small group living. Relationships framed by accountability and responsibility in providing individualised care appear to enable a clear sense of purpose.

Building upon the discussion of the findings reported through out this chapter, a number of practice principles may now be stated:

- Relationships and group interaction should be creatively linked by the actions of keyworkers.

- Time with service users is best considered within the context of a personalised service by small staff teams within small living groups. This will build effective relationships that focus upon the quality of the service user's experience. Expectations and priorities need spelling out here.

- Supervision focusing clearly and consistently upon the quality of the service user's experience will create a sense of purpose in relationships.

- Keyworkers, building relationships in their practice with service users, will usefully:
  1. Promote and cultivate special interests.
  2. Utilise the enabling and supportive role of supervision.
  3. Establish areas of common interest between themselves and service users.

- Effective practice for individualised care will creatively work with the dynamics of small group living:
  1. Providing a personalised 24 hour cover, by keyworkers working as a series of small staff teams.
  2. Building effective individual relationships in the context of the small living group.
  3. Ensuring that tensions between individuals and the group are worked through. Keyworkers have a primary role here.
  4. Focusing upon the quality of user's experience. Clear and consistent supervision is the key to enabling this.
  5. Ensuring clarity in goals and goal attainment. The aims of keyworking should relate to enabling small group living as well as individualising care.

It is recommended that:

- Keyworkers strive to create positive relationships within group living, advocating individual service user need, promoting shared decision making, and working through tensions between individuals and groups.

- A full personalised service is provided on a 24 hour basis with keyworkers working as a series of small staff teams.

- Time spent by keyworkers with service users focuses upon a personalised service provided by the staff team in the context of the group experience.

- Expectations of staff and priorities are defined in conjunction with supervisors and service users. Priorities defined here focus upon the provision of a service by keyworkers and the staff team.

- Supervision focuses clearly and consistently upon the quality of the service user's experience creating a sense of purpose.

3.2. Developing keyworker practice: practice principles: (b) decision making/meeting needs

The findings and discussion in this chapter suggested that the main strengths of keyworking in relation to meeting needs appeared to lie in creating a sense of focus beyond physical care to meet emotional needs. The keyworker role in focusing upon care planning gave a firm sense of structure linking relationships with needs defined and met through joint decision making. Informal day to day involvement of service users in decisions was actively pursued by keyworkers. Keyworkers prioritised tasks in discussion with senior staff and in discussion with service users. Successful links were made with relatives by keyworkers in order to define needs and implement the individual service user's care plan. The support of relatives established a sense of security for the service user.

Keyworking as the main focus in the establishment for care planning, defining and meeting needs and individual decision making in daily living is one occurring throughout the keyworker literature (e.g: Ward, 1987; Sackville, 1979; Pragnell, 1983 and Mallinson, 1989a. Plus in relation to networking and liaison: Cambridge, 1992 and Dant and Gearing, 1990).

Building upon the discussion of the findings reported throughout this chapter, a number of practice principles may now be stated:

- Shared decision making should be established in everyday practice in the keyworker service user relationship.

- Participation should be allied with accountability in the provision of a service of quality by keyworkers.

- Needs should be interpreted through discussions with relatives. The rights of users and the provision of a service are central elements here.

- Supervision should focus upon the quality of service user's experience and promote shared decision making.

- The keyworker should be seen as the coordinator of the care plan. The plan will need to focus upon the quality of the service user's experience.

- Actions that provide for effective decision making in order to meet individual needs in keyworker practice will:
  1. Recognise tensions between the user/keyworker relationship and managerial accountability, thus enabling clarity in hierarchical levels of decision making.
  2. Promote shared decisions between user, keyworker and supervisor.
  3. Interpret needs through discussions with relatives.
  4. Utilise the rights of users as a focus for decision making.
  5. Focus on the provision of a service of quality by keyworkers.

It is recommended that:

- Participative decision making is promoted by keyworkers within living groups.

- The keyworker is seen as the coordinator of the service user's care plan. The plan focuses upon the quality of user's experience.

- Keyworker enable networks and promote effective involvement of relatives.

- Needs are, if appropriate, interpreted through discussions by keyworkers and supervisors with relatives.

- Accountability is formulated within the keyworker/ service user relationship, and in care planning focusing upon everyday practice in the provision of a service of quality.

- Tensions within the user/keyworker relationship and managerial accountability are recognised and talked through. The rights of users will provide a focus for decision making here.

3.3. Developing keyworker practice: practice principles: (c) the role of keyworkers

The findings and discussion in this chapter suggested that sound practice in relation to the role of keyworker appeared to lie in a number of factors. Supervision of quality will promote good practice in day to day events focusing upon individual goal - setting and overall plans for the setting. A clear chain of communication enables decision making and clear boundaries of responsibility. Roles may be divided by agreement between keyworkers and their supervisors so long as there is a clarity in their formulation, and they are subject to review. The dual notion of keyworking and an overall responsibility provides a sense of focus to keyworker systems in relation to the broader task in hand. Relationships linked with accountability provide a firm sense of task for keyworkers.

Building upon the discussion of the findings reported through out this chapter, a small number of practice principles may now be stated:

- Aims and objectives should be established to provide a framework for keyworker roles and tasks and create expectations.
- A notion of accountability of all staff focusing upon role should be established.
- Supervision should be utilised to enable a framework for keyworker roles and tasks, setting standards and expectations.

It is recommended that:

- Aims and Objectives provide a framework for keyworker roles and tasks, setting out expectations of staff and standards to be applied. Individual keyworker effectiveness is promoted through the use of aims and objectives in supervision.
- The task of keyworkers has a clear focus upon the quality of user's experience and clarity in goals and goal attainment. Supervision focuses upon attaining this.
- Maintaining a sense of purpose in all structures within the setting is used to assist clarity in role.
- Care planning structures are used to promote accountability to service users.

- Accountability focusing on role is utilised to achieve clarity in goals and goal attainment.

- Supervision is used to enable a framework for keyworker roles and tasks and promoting shared decision making and accountability, setting standards and expectations.

4. Overall conclusions

The question may now be posed: Does keyworking in residential care for older people contribute towards improved individualised care?

The evidence from both the survey and the researched case studies indicated that structures and systems focusing on individualised care in a group context may be directly linked to keyworker systems. Small group living and keyworking appear, in many cases, to exist together as a dynamic entity. Practice related to both sets of structures is taken by keyworkers on a continuing basis.

The survey indicated that there are differences in staffing arrangements in establishments with keyworkers compared with those without. In establishments with keyworkers, staffing would generally appear to focus more directly upon the quality and continuity of individualised relationships.

Keyworkers undertake a variety of tasks that focus upon individualised care in a group context. They maintain a network of contacts to carry out this. Co-keyworking is practised in a number of establishments enabling cover and a wider dimension to individualised practice.

A high proportion of establishments felt that keyworker systems improved individualised care, relationships, clarity of the residential task, and other aspects of the life of the establishment. Aspects of these that occurred particularly frequently in the survey results were: staff and service users to get to know each other as people; the fulfilment of service users' personal needs; getting to know each other; enhancement of trust; better communication; and a greater knowledge of the needs of the individual. Some problem areas were highlighted, these particularly related to resourcing difficulties and deployment.

The picture painted of the two establishments explored as in depth case studies illustrated the diversity of approaches to individualised care that were possible within differing settings.

The strengths of keyworking relate to the creation of purposeful relationships within the group setting. Successful keyworking links decision making and meeting needs to relationships that individualise care in the context of the staff team as a whole. This is within the broader questions of meeting group needs and group living requirements. Keyworking is a creative base for practice which can be made purposeful and have a sense of focus and structure. The quality of structures (such as care planning and supervision) upon which this is dependent, and how these structures are interpreted is the very weakness of keyworking in that it gives rise to a large amount of individual variability. This is particularly so where quality of individual relationships within structures (supervisor/ keyworker, and keyworker/ service user) interact with quality of interpretation and use of the actual structures themselves.

It is clear that realising excellence in practice will be dependent upon the calibre of the individual keyworker, the formulation of first class systems and structures, and the creation of an ethos of quality. A minimalist view of practice that reduces keyworking to a system of task allocation, rather than promoting quality of care planning, supervision, teamwork and relationships is to be avoided, but in the realities of individual (or collective) practice may often occur. There is thought to be considerable variations within establishments (and between individual keyworkers) as well as between establishments. This lack of consistency is the single most important drawback of the keyworker concept. Whilst varieties of practice may be countenanced between establishments, they should not be countenanced between individuals to the extent that they appear so to do. The effect of this variability upon outcomes of care should not be minimised. Differential quality in relationships and the resulting action in individualising care will result in different effects. The issue here is minimum standards and expectations /requirements which in many instances do not appear to exist or where they may exist are not applied with any degree of rigour.

Practice within structures is heavily dependent upon action taken by particular individuals. The interpretation of action required is often variable. It would appear however, that keyworking in residential establishments for older people as provider settings for care may build relationships and enable group interaction. Keyworking may enable a shared view of priorities between service users and the wider network of care. Care planning linked with keyworker systems may be utilised to give focus and a sense of structure to providing for individual needs. The roles of monitoring and direct service provision appear to be particularly important here. The lack of standards and consistency in expectations must give rise to considerable concern.

This book indicates that keyworking in residential care for older people does contribute towards improved individualised care. Practice here is particularly effective when considered within the broader context of group living and the overall work of the staff team. Its effectiveness is, however, dependent upon the calibre of a broad tapestry of systems and structures (in particular those concerning supervision, evaluation and care planning), how these are utilised within keyworker systems and upon the nature of the individual keyworker/ service user relationship. The weakness of the concept lies in the variability of practice and relationships within establishments when minimum standards and requirements are not defined and/or not applied.

Bibliography

Adams, J. L. (1987), *Conceptual Blockbusting,* Penguin, Harmonsworth.

Adcoc,k M., White, R. and Rowlands, O. (1983), *The Administrative Parent: A Study of the Assumption of Parental Rights and Duties,* BAAF, London.

Ainsworth, F. and Fulcher, L. C. (1981), *Group Care for Children - Concepts and Issues*, Tavistock, London.

Algie, J. (1975a). *Social Values, Objectives and Action*, Kogan Page, London.

Algie, J. (1975b). 'Comment', *Social Work Today,* vol. 6, no. 10, 21 August 1975, Birmingham, p. 289.

Allen-Meares, P. and Lane, B. A. (1987), 'Grounding social work practice in theory: ecosystems', *Social Casework,* October 1987, Family Service America, pp. 515-521.

Anderson, D. (1982), *Social Work and Mental Handicap*, Macmillan, Basingstoke.

Argyris, C. and Schon, D. A. (1974), *Theory in Practice, Increasing Professional Effectiveness*, Jossey-Bass, San Francisco.

Argyris, C. (1964), *Integrating the Individual and The Organisation,* Wiley, New York.

Armstrong, J. (1987), *Staying Active: A Positive Approach in Residential Homes,* Centre for Policy on Ageing, London.

Atherton, J. S. (1989), *Interpreting Residential Life: Values to Practise,* Tavistock/ Routledge, London.

Audit Commission, (1983), *Improving Economy, Efficiency and Effectiveness in Local Government in England and Wales*, Audit Commission, London.

Audit Commission, (1986), *Performance Review in Local Government: A Handbook for Auditors*, Audit Commission, London.

Bailey, D., Boyes, D., Brooks, J., Butterworth, A., Collett, M., Conway, J., Davis, L., Hughes, J., and White, P. (1989), Enabling users to control their own lives, *Social Work Today,* 9 March 1989, London, pp. 18-19.

Baldwin, N. (1990), *The Power to Care in Children's Homes,* Avebury, Aldershot.

Baldwin and Harris (1989), quoted in Elkan and Kelly (1991).

Bamford, T. (1990), *The Future of Social Work*, Macmillan, Basingstoke.
Bartlett, H. M. (1970), *The Common Base of Social Work Practice,* National Association of Social Workers, New York.
BASW (1985), *Report on the Management of Child Abuse*, British Association of Social Workers, Birmingham.
Beardshaw, V. and Towell, D. (1990), *Assessment and Case Management*, Kings Fund, London.
Berseford, P. and Croft, S. (1986a), 'Private care or public services?', *Community Care,* 3-7-86, Wallington, pp. 17-18.
Beresford, P. and Croft, S. (1986b), *Whose Welfare – Private Care or Public Services?,* Brighton Polytechnic.
Beresford, P. and Croft, S. (1987), 'Accountability: getting involved in social services work', *Social Work Today,* 6 April 1987, Birmingham, p. 11.
Berry, J. (1975), *Daily Experience in Residential Life*, Routledge and Kegan Paul, London.
Bettelheim, B. (1974), *A Home for the Heart,* Thames and Hudson, London.
Biddle, B. J. (1979), *Role Theory: Expectations, Identities and Behaviour,* Academic Press, New York.
BIOSS (1974), *Social Services Departments, Developing Patterns of Work and Organisation*, Brunel Institute of Organisation and Social Studies, Heinemann, London.
Bond, M. (1992), 'Time is on our side', *Social Work Today,* 27 February 1992, London, pp. 24-25.
Booth, T., Barritt, A., Berry, S., Martin, D. N., Melotte, C., Phillips, D. (1982), 'A confused mixture', *Community Care,* 2 December 82, Wallington, pp. 12-14.
Booth, T., Barritt, A., Berry, S., Martin, D.N., Melotte, C. and Stone, S. (1982), 'Levels of dependency in local authority homes for the elderly', *Journal of Epidemiology and Community Health,* vol. 36, no. 1, March 1982, pp. 53-57.
Booth, T., Barritt, A., Berry, S., Martin, D. N., and Melotte, C. (1983), 'Dependency in residential homes for the elderly', *Social Policy and Administration,* vol. 17, no. 1, Spring 1983, pp. 46-52.
Booth. T., Bilson, A. and Fowell, I. (1990), 'Staff attitudes and caring practices in homes for the elderly', *British Journal of Social Work,* Oxford, pp. 117-149.
Booth, T. (1985), *Home Truths, Old Peoples Homes and the Outcome of Care,* Gower, Aldershot.
Bowlby, J. (1963), *Child Care and the Growth of Love*, Penguin, Harmondsworth.
Braithwaite, R. (1988), 'Creating a place of solace', *Community Care,* 27 October 1988, Wallington, pp. 22-23.
Brearley, C. P. (1975), *Social Work Ageing and Society,* Routledge and Kegan Paul, London, quoted in Dant et al (1989).
Brearley, C. P. (1982a), *Risk and Ageing*, Routledge and Kegan Paul, London.

Brearley, C. P. (1982b), *Risk and Social Work*, Routledge and Kegan Paul, London.
Brent (1985), *A Child in Trust*, London Borough of Brent.
Bromley, G. (1977), 'Interaction between field and residential social workers', *British Journal of Social Work*, vol. 7, no. 3, pp. 285-299.
Brown, B. J. and Christie, M. M. (1981), *Social Learning Practice in Residential Child Care*, Pergamon Press, Oxford, quoted in Brown. (1986).
Brown, D. and Brearley, P. (1990), 'Homes in a warm climate', *Insight*, 4 July 1990, London. (pp. 24-27)
Brown, B. (1986), *Reliability of the Staff Performance Rating Scale*, Orchard Lodge Studies of Deviancy, vol. 6, no. 1, Winter 1986, London.
Bryman, A. (1988), *Quantity and Quality in Social Research*, Unwin Hyman, London.
Bulmer, M. (1987), *The Social Basis of Community Care*, Allen and Unwin, London, quoted in Dant et al (1989).
Burgess, R. G. (1982), *Field Research: A Sourcebook and Field Manual*, Routledge, London.
Burningham, S. (1983), 'Who makes the rules?', *Social Work Today*, 25 October 1983, Birmingham, pp. 10-11.
Burns, T. and Stalker, G. M. (1961), *The Management of Innovation*, Tavistock, London.
Burt, M. (1985), 'The importance of the team role', *Social Work Today*, 30 September 1985, Birmingham, pp. 16-17.
Burton, J. (1989), Making it work: group living in residential care, *Social Work Today*, 6 June 1989, London, pp. 16-17.
Butrym, Z. T. (1976), *The Nature of Social Work*, Macmillan London.
Cadwallander, M. (1959), 'The cybernetic analysis of change in complex organisations', *American Journal of Sociology*, 65, Chicago, p. 154-7.
Cambridge, P. (1992), 'Case management in community services: organisational responses', *British Journal of Social Work*, vol. 22, October 1992, Oxford University Press, p. 495-517.
Canter and Canter (1979), quoted in Kellaher (1986).
Carnall, C. and Maxwell, S. (1988), *Management: Principles and Policy*, ICSA Publishing, Cambridge.
Carradice, P. (1985), 'The rights and wrongs of rights', *Social Work Today*, 4 November 1985, Birmingham, p. 21.
Caroll, S. J. and Tosi, H. (1973), *Management by Objectives – Allocations and Viewpoints*, Macmillan, New York.
Cassidy, T. (1986), 'Objective setting and evaluation in residential and day care', *Social Work Education*, vol. 5, pp. 22-24.
CCETSW (1973), *Social Work: Residential Work is part of Social Work*, Central Council for Education and Training in Social Work, Paper 3, London.
CCETSW (1992a), *Setting Quality Standards for Residential Child Care*, Central Council for Education and Training in Social Work, London.

CCETSW (1992b), *Residential Child Care in the Diploma in Social Work, Guidance on Knowledge, Values, Skills and Competence,* Central Council for Education and Training in Social Work, London.

Centre for Policy on Ageing (1990), *Community Life: A Code of Practice for Community Care*, CPA, London.

Challis, D. (1985), in Hatch, S. (ed.), *Decentralisation and Care in the Community,* Policy Studies Institute, Discussion Paper No. 10, London.

Challis, D. and Chesterman, J. (1985), A system for monitoring social work activity with the frail elderly, *British Journal of Social Work*, vol. 15, pp. 115-132, quoted in Dant et al (1989).

Challis, D., Darton, R., Johnson, L. and Stone, M. (1988), 'Multi-skilled carers in the community', *Social Work Today*, 4-8-88, London, pp. 13-15.

Challis, D., Darton, R., Johnson, L., Stone, M., Traske, K. and Wall, B. (1989), *Supporting Frail Elderly at Home*, PSSRU University of Kent, Canterbury.

Challis, D. and Davies, B. (1986), *Case Management in Community Care,* Gower, Aldershot.

Checkland, P. (1981), *Systems Thinking, Systems Practice*, Wiley and Sons, Chichester.

Chess, W. A. and Norlin, J. M. (1991), *Human Behaviour and the Social Environment: A Social Systems Model*, Allyn and Bacon, Boston.

Clark, C. L. and Asquith, S. (1985), *Social Work and Social Philosophy, A Guide for Practice,* Routledge and Kegan Paul, Library of Social Work, London.

Clarke, L. (1992), Qualitative research: meaning and language, *Journal of Advanced Nursing,* 17, pp. 243-252.

Clifton Williams, J. (1978), *Human Behaviour in Organisations*, South Western Publishing, Cincinnati.

Clough, R. (1986), 'Staffing of Residential Homes', in Judge, K. and Sinclair, I., *Residential Care for Elderly People*, HMSO, London.

Cohen, B. Z. (1987), 'The ethics of social work supervision revisited', *Social Work (USA),* May-June 1987, pp. 194-196.

Cooper, D. M. and Ball, D. (1987), *Social Work and Child Abuse*, Macmillan Education, Basingstoke.

Cotmore, R., Sinclair, R., Webb, A., and Wistow, G. (1985), 'Five faces of care', *Community Care,* 27 June 1985, Wallington, pp. 15-18.

Counsel and Care (1992), *From Home to a Home*, Counsel and Care, London.

Cronin, A. (1975), 'Comment', *Social Work Today,* 24 July 1975, Birmingham, p. 257.

Crosbie, D. (1983), A role for anyone? A description of social work with the elderly in two area offices, *British Journal of Social Work*, vol. 13, pp,123-148, quoted in Dant et al (1989).

Cyert, R. M. and March, J. G. (1963), *A Behavioral Theory of the Firm*, Wiley New York.

Dalin, P. (1978), *Limits to Educational Change*, Macmillan, London.

Dant, T., Gearing, B., Carley, M., and Johnson, M. (1989), *Keyworkers for Elderly People in the Community: Case Mangers and Care Co-ordinators*, Open University Department of Health and Social Welfare/Policy Studies Institute, Care of Elderly People at Home Project Paper No.6, Milton Keynes.

Dant, T. and Gearing, B. (1990). 'Keyworkers for elderly people in the community: case management and care co-ordinators', *Journal of Social Policy*, vol. 19, no. 3, July 1990, pp. 331-360.

Davies, B. and Knapp, M. (1981), *Old People's Homes and the Production of Welfare*, Routledge and Kegan Paul, London.

Davies, M. (1985), *The Essential Social Worker, A Guide to Positive Practice*, 2nd Edition, Wildwood House, Gower Aldershot.

Davis, L. (1978,) 'Beyond the keyworker concept', *Social Work Today*, 10 January 1978, Birmingham, p. 17.

Davis, L. (1982), *Residential Care: A Community Resource*, Heinemann, London.

Davis, L. (1985), 'When the rules take over', *Social Work Today*, 29 July 1985, Birmingham, p. 19.

DeGreene, K. B. (1981), 'Systems and Psychology', in Open University (1981) *Systems Behaviour*, 3rd edition, Paul Chapman, London. (Reprinted from DeGreene, K. B. (ed.) (1970), *Systems Psychology*, McGraw-Hill.)

DHSS (1976), *Non-Accidental Injury to Children: Area Review Committees*, Department of Health and Social Security, Circular LASSL(76)2/CMO(76)2, London.

DHSS (1979), *Residential Care for the Elderly in London, Social Work Service*, London Region, cited in Lishman, J. (1982), *Developing Services for the Elderly*, Research Highlights in Social Work No 3, University of Aberdeen, Kogan Page, London.

DHSS (1988), *Working Together*, HMSO, London.

Dominelli, L. (1988), *Anti-Racist Social Work*, Macmillan, Basingstoke.

DOH (1990a), *Residential Accommodation for Elderly and for Younger Handicapped People: RA90/2 All Residents in Local Authority, voluntary and Private Homes Year Ending 31-3-90, England*, Department of Health, London.

DOH (1990b), *The Care Programme Approach for People with a Mental Illness Referred to the Specialist Psychiatric Services*, Department of Health, Joint Health /Social Services Circular HC(90)23/LASSL(90)11, London.

DOH/SSI (1989), *Homes are for Living In*, Department of Health/Social Services Inspectorate, HMSO, London.

DOH (1993), *Guidance on Standards for the Residential Care Needs of People with Specific Mental Health Needs*, HMSO, London.

Domoney, L. and Halves (eds.) (1989), *Directory of Practice Examples in Residential Care for Elderly People*, National Institute for Social Work, London.

Douglas, R. and Payne, C. (1980), What happened to the keyworker idea? *Social Work Today*, 21 October 1980, Birmingham, p. 16.

Douglas, R. and Payne, C. (1987), *Learning about Caring, An Introductory Package for Staff Development in Residential and Day Care Work,* National Institute for Social Work, London.
Douglas, R. and Payne, C. (1988) *Organising for Learning*, National Institute for Social Work, London.
Douglas, R., Ettridge, D., Fearnhead, D., Payne, C., Pugh, D., and Sowter, D. (1988), *Helping People Work Together: A Guide to Participative Working Practices*, National Institute for Social Work, Paper 21, London.
Dunham, J. (1980), 'The effects of communication difficulties on social workers', *Social Work Today*, 29 January 1980, Birmingham, pp. 10-12.
Dubois, D., Mockler, B. and Mockler, G. (1984). 'Foster parents as keyworkers/work with natural parents', *Adoption and Fostering,* vol. 8, no. 3, British Association of Adoption and Fostering Agencies, London, pp. 30-33.
Egan, G. (1986), *The Skilled Helper, A Systematic Approach to Effective Helping*, Brooks/Cole Publishing Company, Monterey, California.
Elkan, R. and Kelly, D. (1991), *A Window in Homes: Links between Residential Care Homes and the Community*, Social Care Association, Surbiton.
Elliot, D. (1978), Integrated methods and residential work, *Social Work Today,* 14 February 1978, Birmingham, pp. 11-14.
Elliot, D. (1980), *Some Current Issues in Residential Work: Implications for the Social Work Task*, in Walton and Elliott (1980).
Elliot, D. (1982), A second opinion, *Social Work Today*, 6 April 1982, Birmingham, p. 15.
Ely, P., and Denney, D. (1987), *Social Work in a Multi-Racial Society,* Gower, Aldershot.
Emery, F. E. and Trist, E. L. (1965), 'The causal texture of organisational environments', *Human Relations,* vol. 18, no. 1, February 1965, pp. 21-32.
Evans, D. (1987), 'Getting the balance right', *Community Care,* 11 June 1987, Wallington, p 18-19.
Family Rights Group (1982), *Accountability in Child Care - Which Way Forward?*
Farrar, J. and Tierney, T. (1985), 'Joint evaluation by worker, supervisor and client', *FSU Quarterly,* May 1985, pp. 33-37.
Feak, D. (1982), 'Filling a gap', *Community Care,* 9 September 82, Wallington, pp. 20-21.
Fennell, P. (1986), 'Power-client involvement and drop-in centres, *FSU Quarterly,* July/ August 1986, pp. 24-26.
Ferlie, E., Challis, D. and Davies, B. (1989), *Efficiency-Improving Innovations in Social Care of the Elderly,* Gower, Aldershot.
Ferlie, I., Pahl, J. and Quine, L. (1984). Professional collaboration in services for mentally handicapped people, *Journal of Social Policy,* vol. 13, part 2, Cambridge University Press, Cambridge, pp. 188-202.
Fewster, G. (1979), 'Canada: Residential Adolescent Treatment', in Payne and White (1979).

Fisher, M., March, P., Phillips, D. and Sainbury, E. (1986), *In and Out of Care,* Batsford/BAAF, London.
Fletcher, J. (1985), 'Have You Ever Thought of Living in a Home?', in McDerment and Greengross (1985).
Forrest, A. (1984), *Delegation*, Industrial Society, London.
Francis, W. (1985,) 'Who should carry the can', *Community Care,* 27 June 1985, Wallington, pp. 26-27.
Fulcher, L. C. and Ainsworth, F. (1985), *Group Care Practice with Children,* Tavistock, London.
Gardner, R. (1987), 'Children's participation in care decisions', *Adoption and Fostering,* vol. 11, no. 2, London, pp. 12-14.
Garland, D. S. R. (1987), 'Residential child care workers as primary agents of family intervention', *Child and Youth Care Quarterly,* Human Science Press, pp. 21-34.
Giddens, A. (1979), *Central Problems in Sociological Theory, Action, Structure and Contradiction in Social Analysis,* Macmillan, London.
Gilbert, N. (ed.), (1993), *Researching Social Life*, Sage, London.
Glampson, A. and Goldberg, E. M. (1976), 'Post Seebohm social services: (2) the consumer's viewpoint', *Social Work Today*, vol. 8, no. 6, 9 November 1976, Birmingham, pp. 7-12.
Glastonbury, B. (1975), 'The social worker: "cannon fodder" in the age of admin.?', *Social Work Today*, vol. 6, no. 10, 21 August 1975, Birmingham, pp. 290-292.
Glastonbury, B., Bradley, R., and Orme, J. (1987), *Managing People in the Personal Social Service,* John Wiley and Sons, Chichester.
Glendinning, G. (1986), *A Single Door, Social Work with Families of Disabled Children,* Allen and Unwin, London.
Goffman, E. (1961) ,*Encounters*, Bobbs-Merrill, Indianapolis.
Goldberg, E. M. and Connelly, (1982), *The Effectiveness of Social Care for the Elderly,* Heinemann Educational Books, London.
Goldberg, E. M. and Warburton, R. W. (1979), *Ends and Means in Social Work,* Allen and Unwin, London, quoted in Dant et al (1989).
Goldsmith, J. M. (1977), 'Residential treatment today: the paradox of new premises', *American Journal of Orthopsychiatry,* vol. 46, no. 3, 1976, Jewish Board of Guardians, New York, pp. 453-33, abstract quoted in *Social Work Research and Abstracts,* vol. 13, no. 2, 1977, National Association of Social Workers, New York, p. 70.
Goldstein, H. (1973), *Social Work Practice a Unitary Approach*, University of South Carolina Press, Colombia.
Gostick, C. (1984), 'A Measure of Welfare', *Community Care,*27 September 1984, Wallington, pp. 23-24.
Grant, G., Humphreys, G. and McGrath, M. (1986), *Community Mental Handicap Teams: Theory and Practice*, BIMH Conference Series, Kidderminster.
Gray, B. and Isaacs, B. (1979), *Care of the Mentally Infirm,* Tavistock, London.

Hambleton, R. and Hoggett, R. (1990), *Beyond Excellence: Quality Local Government in the 1990s,* Working paper 85, University of Bristol School of Advanced Urban Studies.

Hamlin, E. R. II and Timberlake, E. M. (1982), 'Peer group supervision for supervisors', *Social Casework, (USA),* February 1982, pp. 82-87.

Hammersley, M., and Atkinson, P., (1983), *Ethnography Principles in Practice*, Tavistock, London.

Hanvey, C. (1987), 'Social work as she is spoke', *Community Care,* 30 April 1987, Wallington, pp. 16-17.

Harris, D. (1975), 'Personal view, tinker, tailor, fieldworker, residential worker', *Social Work Today*, 6 February 1975, Birmingham, p. 693.

Harris, J. and Kelly, D. (1991), *Management Skills in Social Care,* Ashgate, Aldershot.

Hepinstall, D. (1982), 'Management in elderly people's homes', *Community Care,* 27 May 1982, Wallington, pp. 17-20.

Hilgendorf, L. (1981), *Social Workers and Solicitors in Child Care Cases,* HMSO, London.

HMSO (1985), *Social Work Decisions in Child Care*, HMSO/DHSS, London.

HMSO (1989), *The Children Act*, HMSO, London.

HMSO (1989, *Caring for People, Community Care in the Next Decade and Beyond*, HMSO, London.

Hogan, M. (1988), 'Matching a keyworker to the needs of the client', *Social Work Today,* 28-4-88, London, p 27.

Howe, J. (1990), 'The Croxteth Park project', *Social Care Education,* no. 8, Septenber/October 1990, Social Care Association, Surbiton, pp. 21-22.

Hugman, R. (1991), *Power in Caring Professions*, Macmillan Education, Basingstoke.

Hulley, T. (1985), 'Let's give the client responsibility', *Social Work Today,* 6 May 1985, Birmingham, p. 17.

Hunter, D. J. (1988), *Bridging the Gap: Case Management and Advocacy for People with Physical Handicaps*, King Edward's Hospital Fund, London.

Jack, R. (1986), 'The assessment of the elderly mentally ill', *Action Baseline,* Spring 1986, London, pp. 15-18.

Jamieson, B. D. (1973), 'Behavioural problems with management by objectives', *Academy of Management Journal,* September 1973, pp. 496-505.

Johnson, D. (1991), 'Computer care plans make history come to life', *Care Weekly,* 25 October 1991, London, p 12.

Johnson, S. (1981), 'Staff cohesion in residential treatment', *Journal of Youth and Adolescence,* vol. 10, no. 3, June 1981, pp. 221-232.

Johnson, S. (1982), 'Staff cohesion in residential treatment', *Child Care Quarterly,* vol. 11, part 3, Fall 1982, pp. 204-210.

Johnston, S. (1988), 'The Implementation of a Keyworker System', in Mallinson (1988), *Social Care Practice with Elderly Persons*, Social Care Association, Surbiton.

Jones, A., Phillips, M. and Maynard, C. (1992), *A Home from Home, The Experience of Black Residential Projects as Focus of Good Practice,* National Institute for Social Work, London.

Jones, M. (1968), *Beyond the Therapeutic Community, Social Learning and Social Psychiatry*, Yale University Press, New Haven.

Kasushin, A. (1976), *Supervision in Social Work*, Colombia University Press, New York.

Kellaher, L. A. (1986), 'Determinants of quality of life in residential settings for old people', in Judge, K. and Sinclair, I., *Residential Care for Elderly People*, HMSO, London.

Kelly, D. (1987), 'Working towards new relationships for residents and staff, *Social Work Today*, 13 April 1987, Birmingham, p 25.

Kelly, D. and Beck, M. (1990), 'Home front: the power of choice', *Community Care Supplement,* 7 June 1990, Wallington.

Kelsall, J. and McCullough, B. (1988), *Family Work in Residential Child Care: Partnership in Practice,* Boys and Girls Welfare Society, Manchester Free Press, Cheadle.

Khatz, D. and Khan, R. L. (1978), *The Social Psychology of Organisations*, 2nd edition, Wiley, New York.

King, N., Anderson, N. and West, M. A. (1991), 'Organisational innovation in the UK: a case study of perceptions and processes, *Work and Stress,* vol. 5, no. 4, p. 331-339.

Knight, B. and Walker, D. L. (1985), 'Towards a definition of alternatives to institutionalisation', *Gerontologist,* vol. 25, no. 4, August 1985, Washington DC, pp. 358-363.

Knight, J. (1986), 'Transference and counter-transference in social work', *Journal of Social Work Practice,* vol. 2, part 2, May 1986, London, pp. 4-14.

Kossen, S. (1983), *The Human Side of Organisations*, Harper and Row, New York.

Langan, M. and Lee, P. (1989), *Radical Social Work Today*, Unwin Hyman, London.

Latting, S. E. (1986), 'Adaptive Supervision', *Administration in Social Work,* vol. 10, part 1, Spring 1986, New York, pp. 15-23.

Lee, P. and Pitters, D. (1980), 'Radical Residential Child Care: Trojan Horse or Non-runner?', in Brake, M. and Bailey, R. (eds.), *Radical Social Work and Practice*, Edward Arnold, London.

Leigh, A. (1989), 'When a manager's personal style inspires creativity', *Social Work Today*, 21 September 1989, London, pp. 20-21.

Ledger, R. (1980), 'Residential turnover – should you remain at your post?', *Social Work Today*, 17 June 1980, Birmingham, pp. 20-21.

Leininger, M. M. (1985), *Qualitative Research Methodology in Nursing,* Gruene and Stratton, Orlando Florida.

Licket, R. (1961), *New Patterns of Management*, McGraw Hill, New York.

Linehan, T. (1990), 'Memory test', *Care Weekly,* 27 July 1990, London, p. 10.

Lipsky, M. (1980), *Street Level Bureaucracy*, Russell Sage, New York.

Lishman, J. (1982), *Developing Services for the Elderly*, Research Highlights in Social Work No. 3, University of Aberdeen, Kogan Page, London.

Locke, A. E., Shaw, K., Saari, L. and Latham, G. P. (1981), 'Goal setting and task performance, *Psychological Bulletin,* vol. 90, pp. 125-52.

Lockett, M. and Spear, R. (1980), *Organisations as Systems*, Open University Press, Milton Keynes.

Lukes, S. (1974), *Power: a Radical View*, Macmillan, London

MacFarlane, A. (1987), 'Open up the channels of communication', *Social Work Today*, 18 May 1987, London, p. 11.

McDerment, L. and Greengross, S. (1985), *Social Care for Elderly People, An International Perspective,* Social Care Association, Surbiton.

McKay, A., Goldberg, E. M. and Fruin, D. J. (1973), 'Consumers and a social services department', *Social Work Today*, vol. 4, no. 16, 15 November 1973, Birmingham, pp. 486-491.

Mallinson, I. and Best, E. (1987), 'Sharing tasks will mean more client choice', *Social Work Today*, 7 December 87, pp. 12-13.

Mallinson, I. and Citarella, V. (1990), 'Making the perfect match', *Community Care,* 26 April 1990, Wallington, pp. 27-29.

Mallinson, I. and Kelly, D. (1990), 'Keyworking a key factor in case management', *Social Work Today*, 28 June 1990, London, p. 35.

Mallinson, I. (1987), 'Key objectives', *Insight,* 20 November 1987, London, pp. 20-22.

Mallinson, I. (1989a), 'The key to keyworking', *Social Work Today,* 30 March 1989, London, p. 28.

Mallinson, I. (1989b), 'The key to meeting each child's needs', *Social Work Today,* 14 December 1989, London, pp. 16-17.

Mallinson, I. (1989c), 'Sustaining the cornerstones of practice', *Insight,* 7 June 1989 London, pp. 20-21.

Mallinson, I. (1989d), 'The key to economy, efficiency and effectiveness', *Insight,* 9 May 1989, London, pp. 12-13.

Mallinson, I. (1990), *Keyworker: The Case Manager*, (Unpublished paper)

Mallinson, I. (1991), *Under New Management, Guidance on the Transfer of Residential Services,* Social Care Practice Centre, Warwick University, Practice Monograph, Coventry.

Marston, N. and Gupta, H. (1977), 'Interesting the old', *Community Care,* 16 November 1977, Wallington, pp. 26-28.

Megginson, L. C., Mosley, D. C. and Pietri, P. H. Jr. (1986), *Management: Concepts and Applications,* Harper International, New York.

Menzies, E. I. P. (1967), *The Functioning of Social Systems as a Defence Against Anxiety,* Tavistock, London.

Merton, R. (1968), *Social Theory and Social Structure*, Free Press, New York.

Mescon, M. H., Albert, M. and Khedouri, F. (1981), *Management: Individual and Organisational Effectiveness,* Harper and Row, London.

Meteyard, B. (1984), 'Turning theory into practice', *Community Care,* 16 February 1984, London, pp. 27-28.
Meteyard, B. (1986), *Keyworker Shop*, Local Government Training Board, Luton.
Meteyard, B. (1987), 'Keyworker', in *In Practice II,* Papers given at Special Interest Workshops, SCA Annual Seminar 1986 Harrogate, Social Care Association, Surbiton.
Meteyard, B. (1990), *Community Care Keyworker Manual*, Longman Consumer Services, Harlow.
Meyer, E. (1986), *A Study of Organisational Reform: an Examination of the Impact of Organisational Structure on Staff Attitudes Within a Residential Setting for Mentally Retarded Persons*, Brandeis Phd, February 1986, abstract in *Social Work Research and Abstracts,* vol. 22, 1986, National Association of Social Workers, New York, p. 42.
Miller, E. J. and Gwynne, G. V. (1972), *A Life Apart*, Tavistock, London.
Millham, S., Bullock, R., Hosie, K. and Haak, M. (1985), *Children Lost in Care, The Family Contact of Children in Care*, Gower, Aldershot.
Moore, J. (1985), *The ABC of Child Abuse Work*, Gower, Aldershot.
Morris, R. (1981), 'Food for thought', *Community Care,* 8 October 1981, Wallington, pp. 14-16.
Morrison, T. (1986), 'Teamwork: beyond the sum of its individuals, *Community Care,* 4 September 1986, Wallington, pp. 26-28.
Moser, C. A. and Kalton, G. (1971), *Survey Methods in Social Investigation,* Heinemann Educational, London.
Mullender, A. (1990), 'Groupwork in residential settings for elderly people, *Groupwork,* vol. 3, no. 3, p. 286-301.
NCVO (1984), *Clients' Rights, Report of a Working Party,* National Council for voluntary Organisations, London.
Neill, J. E., Fruin, D., Goldberg, E. M. and Warburton, R. W. (1973), 'Reactions to integration', *Social Work Today,* vol. 4, no. 15, 1 November 1973, Birmingham, pp. 458-465.
Neill, et al (1988), quoted in Elkan and Kelly(1991).
Neill, J., Sinclair, I., Gorbach, P. and Williams, J. (1988), *A Need for Care? Elderly Applicants for Local Authority Homes*, Avebury Gower, Aldershot.
Ovretveit, J. (1987), 'Aspects of Community Mental Handicap Team Management and Organisation', in Grant, G., Humphreys, S. and Mc Grath, M. (1987), *Community Mental Handicap Teams: Theory and Practice,* BIMH Conference Series, Kidderminster.
NISW (1982), *Social Workers: Their Roles and Tasks (The Barclay Report),* National Institute of Social Work, London.
NISW (1988), *Residential Care, A Positive Choice, Report of the Independent Review of Residential Care*, chaired by Gillian Wagner, National Institute of Social Work, London.

Onyett, S. (1992), *Case Management in Mental Health*, Chapman and Hall, London.
Open University (1985), *T244 Managing in Organisations,* Open University Press, Milton Keynes.
Open University Systems Group (1981), *Systems Behaviour*, Paul Chapman, London.
Packman, J., Randall, J., and Jacques, N. (1986). *Who Needs Care? Social Work Decisions about Children,* Blackwell, Oxford.
Parker, R. A. (1988), 'Children', in Wagner (1988).
Parsons, T. and Shils, E. A. (ed.) (1951), *Towards a General Theory of Action,* Harvard University Press, Cambridge, Massachusetts.
Parsons, T. (1951), *The Social System*, Free Press, Glencoe.
Parsons, T. (1964), 'A Sociological Approach to the Theory of Organisations', in Parsons, T., *Structure and Process in Modern Societies,* Free Press, Glencoe.
Payne, C. and Douglas, R. (1983), 'Key relationship', *Social Work Today,* 7 June 1983, Birmingham, p. 23.
Payne, C. and Scott, T. (1982), *Developing Supervision of Teams in Field and Residential Social Work*, National Institute for Social Work, Paper 12, London.
Payne, C. J. and White, K. J. (1979), *Caring for Deprived Children,* Croom Helm, London.
Perring, C. (1992), 'Home on the range', *Social Work Today*, London, pp. 19-21.
Pettes, D. E. (1979), *Staff and Student Supervision*, National Institute for Social Work, London.
Phillips, D. R., Vincent, J. and Blacksell, S. (1989), *Home from Home? Private Residential Care for Elderly People,* University of Sheffield Joint Unit for Social Services Research, Sheffield.
Phillips, J. (1986), 'Tools of care: planning and managing the care environment', *Social Work Education,* vol. 5, part 2, Summer 1986, pp. 16-19.
Pincus, A. and Minahan, A. (1973), *Social Work Practice: Model and Method,* Peacock, Itaska.
Plank, M. (1982), *Teams for Mentally Handicapped People*, Enquiry Paper 10, The Campaign for Mentally Handicapped People, London.
Pope, P. (1982), 'A new approach', *Community Care,* 2 December 1982, Wallington, pp. 18-19.
Quine, L. and Pahl, J. (1989), *Stress and Coping in Families Caring for a Child with Severe Mental Handicap: A Longitudinal Study,* University of Kent Canterbury.
Raman, S. and Sayce, L. (1992), *Policy changes - Obstacles and Opportunities for collective Users Involvement*, Unpublished paper.

RCA/BASW (1976), 'How can residential and field social workers co-operate?', *Social Work Today*, 2 September 1976, Birmingham, pp. 346-348.

RCA (1976), 'The relationship between field and residential work', *Residential Social Work,* vol. 16, no. 9, September 1976, RCA, London, pp. 235-238.

RCA (1978), *Heads and Hearts*, Residential Care Association, Surbiton.

RCA (1983), 'The keyworker, a special report', *Horizon,* no. 8, August 1983, Residential Care Association, Surbiton.

RCA (1984), 'The keyworker reviewed: a working paper', *Horizon,* no. 16 September 1984, Residential Care Association, Surbiton.

Reading, H. F. (1977), *A Dictionary of the Social Sciences*, Routledge and Kegan Paul, London.

Redding, D. (1991), 'The key to success, inside the NHS and the Community Care Act', *Community Care,* 28 March 1991, Wallington, p. vi.

Renshaw, J., Hampson, R., Thomason, C., Darton, R., Judge, K. and Knapp, M. (1988), *Care in The Community: The First Steps*, Gower, Aldershot.

Rice, A. K. (1963), *The Enterprise and Its Environment*, Tavistock, London.

Richards, K. (1987), 'Accountability for care: we need a comprehensive approach', *Social Work Today*, 6 April 1987, Birmingham, p. 10.

Riordan, J., Bramhall, B. and Backhouse, T. (1988), 'Teamwork to serve the elderly', *Health Service Journal,* 19 May 1988, London, pp. 564-566.

Rivlin, M. (1983), 'Reacting to power', *Social Work Today,* 2 August 1983, Birmingham, p. 21.

Roberts, G. (1989), 'All under one roof', *Community Care,* 27 August 1989, supplement 'Inside Interagency Work', Wallington, pp. v-vi.

Rock, B. D. (1987), 'Goal and outcome in social work practice', *Social Work (USA),* September – October 1987, pp. 393-398.

Rodway, S. (1979), 'The concept of the keyworker: is it "pie and the sky"? An employer's viewpoint', *Social Work Service,* 19 March 1979, Department of Health and Social Security, London, pp. 45-47.

Rodway, S. (1981), 'Love is not love which alters when it alteration finds', *Community Care,* 12 March 1981, Wallington, pp. 12-14.

Roethisberger and Dickson (1939), in Silverman (1970).

Ross, S. and Bilson, A. (1989), *Social Work Management and Practice: Systems Principles,* Jessica Kingsley, London.

Rowbottom, et al (1974), see BIOSS (1974).

Rowe, J., Cain, H., Hundleby, M. and Keane, A. (1984), *Long Term Foster Care,* Batsford/BAAF.

Sackville, A. (1979), The concept of the keyworker: a challenge to traditional thinking, *Social Work Service,* 19 March 1979, Department of Health and Social Security, London, pp. 40-44.

Savage, A. (1985), quoted in Challis, Darton, Johnson and Stone (1988).

Sainsbury, E. (1989), 'Participation and Paternalism', in Shardlow (1989).

Scott, M. (1984), 'Who Calls the Tune?', *Social Work Today*, 16 April 1984, Birmingham, p. 17.
Scottish Office (1993a), *Another Kind of Home, A Review of Residential Care,* The Social Work Services Inspectorate for Scotland, HMSO, Edinburgh.
Scottish Office (1993b), *Statistical Bulletin, January 1993*, The Scottish Office Social Work Services Group, Edinburgh.
Scrutton, S. (1986), ' "I don't like to complain dear" ', *Community Care,* 4 December 1986, Wallington, p 20-21.
SCA/BASW (1987), *Review and Prospect: 10 Years of Keyworking*, unpublished report, Social Care Association, Surbiton.
SCA (1986), 'The keyworker revisited', *Social Work Today,* 17 March 1986, London, p. 25.
SCA (1988), *The Social Care Task,* Social Care Association, Surbiton.
SCA (1990a), *Action Checklist for Anti-Racist Practice in Social Care,* Social Care Association, Surbiton.
SCA (1990b), *Night Care Assistants, Summary of Main Issues Generated in the SCA Annual Seminar,* unpublished document, Social Care Association, Surbiton.
SCA (1991), *Keyworking in Social Care, an Introductory Guide*, Social Care Association, Surbiton.
SCA (1992a), *The Lost Potential*, SCA Education, Coventry.
SCA (1992b), *Giving Good Care: An Introductory Guide for Care Assistants,* SCA Education/ Help the Aged, Surbiton.
SCA (1992c), *Managing the Crisis of Closure, A Good Practice Guide for Residential care*, Social Care Association, Surbiton.
SCA (1993a), *The Social Care Task: Improving the Quality of Life,* Social Care Association, Surbiton.
SCA (1993b), *21 Rights for Care Assistants*, Birmingham and Area Branch, Social Care Association, Birmingham.
SCA (1993c), *Communication Begins at Home*, SCA Education, Surbiton.
Seebohm Report (1968), *Report of The Committee On Local Authority and Allied Social Services*, HMSO, London.
Selzenick, P. (1948), 'Foundations of the theory of organisations', *American Sociological Review,* vol. 13, no. 1, pp. 25-35.
Selzenick, P. (1949), *TVA and the Grass Roots*, California University Press, Berkeley.
Senior, B. (1989), 'Residential Care: What Hope for the Future?', in Langan and Lee (1989).
Shardlow, S. (1989), *The Values of Change in Social Work,* Tavistock/Routledge, London.
Shaw, I. F. (1984), 'Literature review: consumer evaluations of the personal social services, *British Journal of Social Work*, vol. 14, no. 3, June 1984, Oxford, pp. 277-284.
Shenker, B. (1982), 'Is success a dirty word?', *Social Work Service,* no. 30, Summer 1982, p. 36-38.

Siddiqui, S. (1991), 'Ways to shelter from the strain', *Care Weekly,* 19 April 1991, pp. 10-11.

Sills, P. (1988), 'The learning curve', *Care Weekly,* 12 August 1988, p. 10.

Silverman, D. (1970), *The Theory of Organisations*, Heinemann London.

Sinclair, R. (1983), 'The nature of decisions taken at reviews', *Adoption and Fostering,* vol. 7, no. 4, pp. 52-57.

Sinclair, R. (1984), *Decision Making in Statutory Reviews on Children in Care,* Gower, Aldershot.

Sinclair and Payne (1989), quoted in Elkan and Kelly (1991).

SSI (1989), *Doing it Better Together, A Report of Developments in Four Locations to Establish Local Procedures for Multidisciplinary Assessment of the Needs of Elderly People*, Social Services Inspectorate, Department of Health, London.

SSI (1991), *Assessment Systems and Community Care*, Social Services Inspectorate, Department of Health, London.

SSI (1993), *Evaluating Performance in Child Protection, A framework for the inspection of local authority social services practice and systems*, Department of Health, HMSO, London.

SSI/SWSG (1991), *Care Management and Assessment: Manager's Guide,* Department of Health, Social Services Inspectorate, HMSO, London.

Stein, M. and Carey, K. (1986), *Leaving Care*, Basil Blackwell, Oxford.

Stevenson, O. and Smith, J. (1975?), *The Implementation of Section 56 of the Children Act 1975,* unpublished research report, quoted in HMSO (1985).

Sutton, C. (1979), *Psychology for Social Workers and Counsellors: An Introduction*, Routledge and Kegan Paul, London.

Taylor (1913), in Silverman (1970).

Taylor, J. (1985), 'Meresworth, Home within a Home', in McDerment and Greengross (1985).

Tavener, P. (1989), Ideas in action: supervision and the nature of the organisation, *Social Work Education,* vol. 8, no. 2, Spring 1989, pp. 25-28.

Thoburn, J. (1986), Quality control in child care, *British Journal of Social Work*, vol. 16, p. 543-556.

Thomas, N. (1981), 'Design, Management and Resident Dependency in Old People's Homes', in Goldberg, E. M. and Connelly, N. (1981), *Evaluative Research in Social Care*, Henemann, London.

Thomas, R. (1975), 'Changing and Improving Educational Systems and Institutions', in Hughes, M. (ed.) (1975), *Administering Education: International Challenge,* Athlone Press, New York.

Tosi, H. L. and Carroll, S. J. (1968), 'Managerial reaction to management by objectives', *Academy of Management Journal,* vol. 11, December 1968, pp. 415-426.

Tossell, D., and Webb, R. (1986), *Inside the Caring Services*, Edward Arnold, London.

Townsend, P. (1962), *The Last Refuge*, Routledge and Kegan Paul, London.

Trist, E. L. et al (1963), *Organisational Choice*, Tavistock, London.

Truax, C. B. and Carkhuff, R. R. (1967), *Towards Effective Counselling and Psychotherapy*, Aldine, Chicago.
Unwin, H. (1987), 'Some Research Concerning General Management Skills', in Sutton, C. (1987), *A Handbook of Research for the Helping Professions,* Routledge and Kegan Paul, London.
Vernon, J. and Fruin, D. (1986), *In Care: A Study of Social Work Decision Making,* National Children's Bureau, London.
Wagner, (1988), *Residential Care: A Positive Choice, Report of the Independent Review of Residential Care*, NISW/HMSO, London.
Walker, P. (1980), 'In care – the facts of life, *Community Care,* 30 October 1980, Wallington, p. 19-22.
Walton, R. G. and Elliott, D. (1980), *Residential care, A Reader in Current Theory and Practice,* Pergamon Press, Oxford.
Ward, L. (1978), 'The keyworker concept', *Social Work Today*, 13 June 1978, Birmingham, p. 1.
Ward, P. (1980), *Quality of Life in Residential Care*, Personal Social Services Council, London.
Webb, E. J., Campbell, D. T., Schwartz, R. D. and Sechrest, L. (1966), *Unobtrusive Measures: Nonreactive Research in The Social Sciences,* Rand McNally, Chicago.
Wendelken, C. (1983), *Children In and Out of Care*, Heinemann Educational, London.
Westheimer, I. J. (1977), *The Practice of Supervision in Social Work, A Guide for Supervisors*, Ward Lock Educational, London.
Wetzel, H. (1986), 'Local authorities should involve parents and young people in case conferences', *Foster Care,* part 47, September 1986, pp. 86-87.
White, K. J. (1979), 'United Kingdom: Independent Long Stay Children's Home', in Payne and White (1979).
Whitehouse, A., Crine, A., and Murray, N. (1982), 'Thereby hangs a tale', *Community Care,* 2 December 1982, Wallington, pp. 14-18.
Wilcocks et al (1982), quoted in Elkan and Kelly (1991).
Wilkins, D. and Hughes, B. (1987), 'Residential care of elderly people: the consumers' views', *Ageing and Society,* vol. 7, part 2, June 1987, pp. 175-201.
Willcocks, D., Peace, S. and Kellaher, L. (1987), *Private Lives in Public Places, A Research-Based Critique of Residential Life in Local Authority Old People's Homes*, Tavistock London.
Williams, D. (1980), 'Positive Care for the Elderly', in Walton and Elliott (1980).
Wiseman, V. and Potter, P. (1989), 'Net curtains and flowers', *Social Work Today*, 22 June 1989, London, pp. 15-17.
Woodcock, M. (1979), *Team Development Manual*, Gower, Aldershot.
Woolrych, R. (1987), 'Is management the answer to problems facing CHMTs?', *Social Work Today* 7 September 1987, London, pp. 8, 9.

Younghusband, E. (1978), *Social Work in Britain: 1950-1975*, George Allen and Unwin, London.

Appendix A
Questionnaire extracts

The relevant parts of the census questionnaire that relate to this study are given below:

4. Does your establishment have arrangements for small living groups?

   Yes ☐

   No ☐

   If Yes, please give details:

   Number of groups Size of groups

5. How many permanent residents are there in your establishment:

	White?	Black?	Other?	(Please specify)
Male?				
Female?				

6. How many full time staff (ie more than 30 hours per week) do you have?

   White? Black? Other? (Please specify)

   Male?

   Female?

6a. Please give a brief breakdown of the grades and structure.

7. How many part time care staff (less than 30 hours per week)?

7a. Please give numbers of these doing less than 10 hours per week:

White? Black? Other? (Please specify)

Male?

Female?

7b. Please give numbers of these doing 10-20 hours per week:

White? Black? Other? (Please specify)

Male?

Female?

7c. Please give numbers of these doing over 20 but under 30 hours per week:

White? Black? Other? (Please specify)

Male?

Female?

11. Do you have a "keyworker" system in your establishment? (Note in the following questions the term "keyworker" includes "linkworker", "attached worker", "specials" etc.)

Yes ☐

No ☐

If Yes:

11a. What term is used?

12. What tasks do "keyworkers" undertake? Please list in order of importance (i.e. 1 is the most important, 10 is the least important).

    Assessment of residents
    Counselling
    Physical Care
    Admissions
    Advocating resident's needs
    Recording
    Arranging activities
    Arranging individual outings
    Supporting daily living
    Other (please specify)

13. How many residents are allocated to each "keyworker"?

17. How do you match residents and keyworkers?

18. What factors should be taken into account in matching?

19. What other professionals do "keyworkers" have regular contact with? (ie. at least once every two months)

    General Practitioners
    Field Social Workers
    District Nurse
    Chiropodist
    Religious leaders
    Other (please specify)

20. Do "Keyworkers" practice co-keyworking at all? (e.g. they are formally paired or work together in teams)?

    Yes ☐

    No ☐

    If Yes, please give details:

22. In your view do "keyworker" systems improve

individualised care?

Yes ☐

No ☐

If Yes, please give details:

Relationships?

Yes ☐

No ☐

If Yes, please give details:

Clarity of the residential task?

Yes ☐

No ☐

If Yes, please give details:

Other aspects of the life of the establishment?

Yes ☐

No ☐

If Yes, please give details:

23. Please give any other comments that you feel might be helpful.

24. This questionnaire is fully confidential and the analysis of results will not mention individual establishments by name. If your establishment would, however, be prepared to be approached for further research (concerning consumer and staff views) to be carried out, please give the address and a contact telephone number below:

Appendix B
Overall characteristics of the census and of the survey of establishments with keyworkers

This appendix outlines the characteristics of the survey of establishments with keyworkers that relate to sector and size of establishments and occurrence of small group living arrangements. This is carried out in relation to the overall data of the census of all residential establishments for older people in Birmingham and the Black country.

1. Sector and size of establishments

According to information prepared by the Government Statistical Office, (DOH, 1990a) in England 71.4% of establishments for older people are in the private sector. This may be compared with 68% in the geographical area that formed the census. 20.8% of establishments in England are in the statutory sector compared with 25% in the census. These differences may be due to the industrial urban nature of the area. The voluntary sector figures are 7% Birmingham and the Black country and 7.8% for the whole of England.

Comparable figures for Scotland in 1990 are given by the Scottish Office (1993b); 43.4% of establishments were in the statutory sector, 35.1% private and 21.5% in the voluntary sector.

Considerable variations in size of establishments existed within the census. The average size of 24 service users (Table 6.1) may be compared with that in England as a whole for the same year (20 service users) and Metropolitan Districts in England (22.8 service users).(DOH, 1990a) In Scotland the average size of establishments was 28 service users (Scottish Office, 1993b)

The validity of grouping establishments into small ones (up to 30 service users) and large ones (those with 31 or more service users) is borne out by DOH, (1990a); and Scottish Office, (1993b). There is a clear national skewing in England and Scotland of local authority establishments to 30+ service users and private sector establishments to less than 30 residents. In the census this was also the case (figure 6.2). There were also differences in size between establishments with keyworkers and those without. All these variations are summarised in table B.1.

Keyworker systems were more likely to occur in large establishments (32 out of 37 <86%>); smaller establishments were less likely to operate keyworker systems (occurrence = 26 out of 65 ie. 40%).

Table B.1
Keyworkers and size of establishments in the census

	Small	Large	Total
No. of establishments with keyworkers (n=58)	26 (40%)	32 (86%)	58 (57%)
Ave. size: no. of users.	18	40	30
No. of establishments without keyworkers (n=44)	39 (60%)	5 (14%)	44 (43%)
Ave. size: no. of users.	14	45	17
Total no. census establishments (n=58)	65 (100%)	37 (100%)	102 (100%)
Ave. size: no. of users.	15	41	24

% of total number of establishments responding in the census

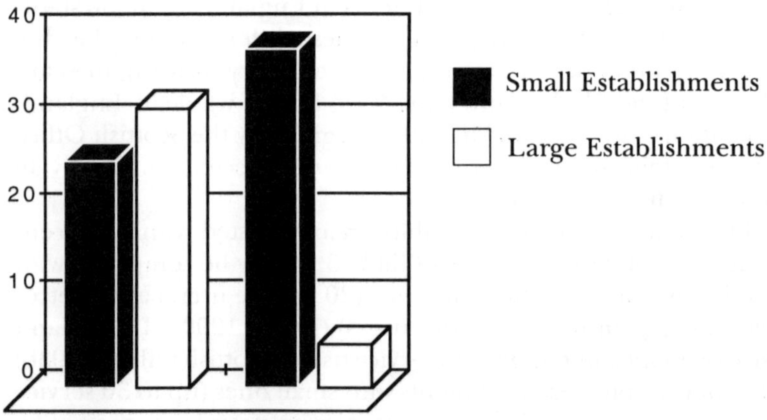

Figure B.1 Keyworkers and size of establishments

Size of establishments in the survey appeared to be a function of the sector as much as whether keyworkers existed or not. This is illustrated by Figure B.2.

*Number of service users in each category of **establishment** (Expressed as mean within each category)*

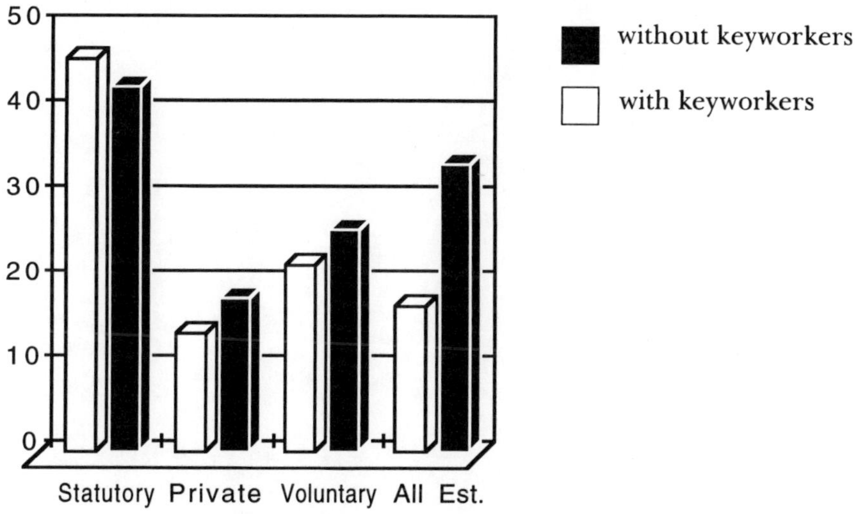

Figure B.2 Mean number of service users in census

2. Small group living

23 residential establishments (23%) in the census made arrangements for small living groups. 5 (42%) of the voluntary establishments 6 (11%) of the private establishments and 17 (46%) of the statutory establishments made such arrangements.

Only 3 establishments without keyworkers had small living groups. Thus 34% of establishments with keyworkers made arrangements for small living groups. 87% of all establishments with small group provision had keyworkers. None of these were in the voluntary sector and only 4 (27%) occurred in the private sector (all of these in smaller establishments).

Thus small group living appeared particularly as a statutory sector phenomena. Of the survey of establishments with keyworkers, 14 out of 29 (48%) large statutory establishments had small group living, similarly, 2 out of 6 (33%) small statutory establishments.

In contrast, comments from small private sector establishments (eg. "None of this questionnaire is applicable as we are a small home that acts as a family; staff are in constant communication") and the lower average size of smaller establishments in the private sector (an average of 14 service users compared with 18/19 service users elsewhere) may indicate that in many cases splitting up living groups was not seen as appropriate in private sector establishments.

Appendix C
Interview checklist and sequence

Relationships

- Nature of keyworker/ service user relationships
- Relationship between keyworking and small living groups:
  - individual needs/choice in a group context
  - commonality of experience of residents
- How are keyworkers matched to service users?
  - criteria
  - methods used
- Practice of co-keyworking

Decision Making/Meeting Needs

- Tasks undertaken by keyworkers
- How tasks are prioritised and carried out
- Networks: Other professionals keyworkers have regular contact with
- Limitations of the role of keyworkers
- Authority of keyworkers,
  - responsibility and
  - accountability
- How are the needs of service users met?

Effect of Keyworker System

- Effect on individualised care
- Effect on relationships
- Do keyworker systems clarify the residential task?